Craving Control: A Guide to Overcoming Food Urges, Shedding Pounds, and Boosting Vitality

By

Calvin M. Duncan

Table of Contents

Chapter One
Introduction

•*The Incidence of Obesity*

The incidence of obesity, characterized by the excessive accumulation of body fat, has risen dramatically over the past few decades, evolving into a global health crisis. This surge in obesity rates is a multifaceted phenomenon influenced by a complex interplay of genetic, environmental, cultural, and behavioral factors. In this chapter, we delve into the drivers behind the incidence of obesity, exploring its prevalence, trends, and the contributing factors that have propelled it to epidemic proportions.

The prevalence of obesity has reached alarming levels worldwide. According to the World Health Organization (WHO), global obesity rates have nearly tripled since 1975. In 2016, more than 1.9 billion adults were overweight, of which over 650 million were classified as obese. Similarly, childhood obesity rates have also risen significantly, with an estimated 41 million children under the age of five being overweight or obese in 2016.

The trajectory of these trends is cause for concern. Left unchecked, the incidence of obesity is projected to continue its upward spiral, posing substantial health, economic, and societal challenges in the years to come.

Genetics play a significant role in an individual's predisposition to obesity. Research has shown that genetics can influence metabolism, hunger regulation, and the body's response to dietary and exercise interventions. However, genetic factors alone cannot account for the rapid increase in obesity rates observed in recent decades.

While genetics may set the stage for an individual's susceptibility to obesity, environmental and behavioral factors ultimately play a pivotal role in determining whether those genetic predispositions are expressed.

The modern environment has undergone significant changes that have contributed to the incidence of obesity. Increased urbanization, technological advancements, and changes in food production and distribution have created an environment that promotes sedentary behaviors and easy access to energy-dense, nutrient-poor foods.

The "obesogenic" environment encourages overeating and discourages physical activity. Highly processed foods that are high in sugars, unhealthy fats, and additives are readily available and often cheaper than fresh, nutritious alternatives. Additionally, the ubiquity of fast food outlets and the promotion of large portion sizes contribute to excessive calorie consumption.

Sociocultural factors also play a pivotal role in the incidence of obesity. Cultural norms and attitudes towards body image can influence eating behaviors and the perception of an ideal body size. In some cultures, being overweight is associated with wealth and prosperity, leading to cultural acceptance of larger body sizes.

Media and advertising play a substantial role in shaping societal beauty ideals and influencing consumer behavior. The portrayal of thinness as the standard of beauty in media can contribute to body dissatisfaction and the adoption of unhealthy weight loss practices.

Individual behaviors are at the heart of the obesity epidemic. Poor dietary choices, such as consuming high-calorie, low-nutrient foods and excessive sugar-sweetened beverages, contribute to calorie surplus. Sedentary behaviors, driven by technology and urbanization, further compound the problem.

Lack of physical activity is a significant factor. Modern lifestyles often involve prolonged periods of sitting, whether it's at a desk, in front of a screen, or during commutes. The decline in physical activity, coupled with the consumption of energy-dense foods, leads to an imbalance between calorie intake and expenditure, resulting in weight gain.

The incidence of obesity is not evenly distributed across populations. Individuals from lower socioeconomic backgrounds often face higher rates of obesity due to limited access to fresh, nutritious foods and fewer opportunities for physical activity. These disparities can create a cycle where obesity exacerbates social and economic challenges, as health issues can limit educational and occupational opportunities.

Childhood experiences play a crucial role in shaping future health outcomes. Poor nutrition and lack of physical activity during childhood can set the stage for obesity later in life. Factors such as maternal nutrition, infant feeding practices, and exposure to unhealthy food environments contribute to the early development of obesity risk.

The incidence of obesity is a multifaceted issue with a complex web of contributing factors. Genetics, environment, culture, behavior, and socioeconomic status all play interconnected roles in driving the obesity epidemic. Addressing this crisis requires a comprehensive approach that involves policy changes, education, and the cultivation of a health-promoting environment.

By understanding the various factors driving the incidence of obesity, we can develop targeted interventions that address the root causes of the problem. As individuals, communities, and societies, we have the power to reverse this trend and create a healthier future for generations to come.

•*The Consequences of the Obesity Epidemic*

In recent decades, the world has witnessed a rapid and alarming rise in obesity rates, giving rise to what is now often referred to as the "obesity epidemic." This global health crisis has far-reaching consequences that extend beyond physical health, impacting various facets of individuals' lives and straining healthcare systems, economies, and societies. In this chapter, we delve into the multifaceted consequences of the obesity epidemic and shed light on the urgent need to address this pressing issue.

One of the most direct and immediate consequences of the obesity epidemic is the burden it places on healthcare systems. Obesity is a major risk factor for numerous chronic diseases, including type 2 diabetes, cardiovascular disease, hypertension, and certain types of cancer. These conditions require ongoing medical attention, medications, and sometimes invasive interventions, all of which drive up healthcare costs significantly.

The obesity-related diseases also lead to a decreased quality of life for affected individuals. Conditions such as joint pain, limited mobility, and shortness of breath can greatly reduce one's ability to engage in daily activities and enjoy life to the fullest. The need for medical care and lifestyle adaptations can lead to emotional distress, further impacting mental health and overall well-being.

The economic consequences of the obesity epidemic are substantial and multifaceted. Healthcare expenditures related to obesity and its associated diseases place a considerable strain on national and global healthcare budgets. Treating obesity-related conditions requires significant resources, from hospital stays to medications and surgeries.

Moreover, the economic impact extends to productivity losses in the workforce. Individuals with obesity may face absenteeism due to health issues or reduced productivity due to limited mobility and chronic conditions. This not only affects individual income but also impacts employers and the economy at large.

Obesity can take a profound toll on individuals' mental and emotional well-being. The stigma associated with being overweight or obese can lead to feelings of shame, low self-esteem, and social isolation. Negative stereotyping and discrimination can exacerbate these feelings, creating a vicious cycle where emotional distress leads to overeating or unhealthy coping mechanisms.

Depression and anxiety are common among individuals with obesity, partly due to the psychosocial challenges they face. The emotional burden of dealing with weight-related issues can contribute to mental health disorders, further compromising individuals' overall quality of life.

The obesity epidemic also intersects with social and cultural dimensions, influencing perceptions of beauty, self-worth, and success. Society's emphasis on thinness as an ideal can lead to body dissatisfaction and disordered eating behaviors among individuals, contributing to a complex interplay between societal norms, personal identity, and body image.

Childhood obesity, in particular, has societal implications. Obese children are at a higher risk of experiencing bullying and social exclusion, which can have lasting psychological effects. The impact on children's health sets the stage for a lifelong struggle with weight-related issues, perpetuating the cycle of the obesity epidemic into the next generation.

The obesity epidemic also has environmental implications. The production and consumption of high-calorie, low-nutrient foods contribute to resource depletion, greenhouse gas emissions, and deforestation. The demand for these types of foods places stress on agricultural systems, perpetuating a cycle that affects not only human health but also the health of the planet.

Addressing the consequences of the obesity epidemic requires a comprehensive and collaborative approach. Governments, healthcare systems, communities, and individuals all play a role in reversing this trend. Education about healthy eating, physical activity, and body positivity is crucial. Access to nutritious foods and safe spaces for physical activity must be prioritized, especially in underserved communities.

Promoting a culture of health and well-being involves destigmatizing obesity and encouraging open conversations about body image and mental health. Effective policies that regulate the marketing of unhealthy foods to children, improve food labeling, and promote active lifestyles are vital components of the solution.

In conclusion, the consequences of the obesity epidemic are far-reaching and impact various aspects of our lives. Beyond the immediate health concerns, the economic, psychological, and societal burdens are substantial. Addressing this issue requires collective efforts to create an environment that supports healthy choices and empowers individuals to take charge of their well-being. By working together, we can mitigate the consequences of the obesity epidemic and pave the way for a healthier future.

•*The Importance of Addressing Obesity and Weight Loss*

Obesity, a condition characterized by excessive body fat accumulation, has become a global epidemic with far-reaching consequences. Beyond aesthetic concerns, obesity poses serious threats to physical health, mental well-being, and overall quality of life. In this chapter, we explore the significance of addressing obesity and the vital role that weight loss plays in promoting individual and societal wellness.

The rise of obesity in recent decades is alarming. A sedentary lifestyle, coupled with easy access to calorie-dense foods, has contributed to an increase in obesity rates across the world. Obesity is linked to a host of health issues, including type 2 diabetes, cardiovascular disease, hypertension, certain types of cancer, and musculoskeletal problems. The excess weight places strain on vital organs and systems, ultimately diminishing their function and increasing the risk of chronic conditions.

Obesity doesn't merely affect physical health; it also has profound psychological and emotional implications. Individuals with obesity often face stigma, discrimination, and negative stereotyping. This social pressure can lead to low self-esteem, anxiety, depression, and a diminished sense of self-worth. The cycle of emotional distress can further fuel overeating and unhealthy eating habits, creating a feedback loop that perpetuates obesity and its associated challenges.

The consequences of obesity extend beyond personal health. The economic burden of obesity is substantial, straining healthcare systems, workplace productivity, and overall societal resources. Medical costs associated with obesity-related diseases place a heavy financial burden on individuals, families, and healthcare providers. Additionally, reduced productivity and increased absenteeism in the workforce further compound the economic impact.

Addressing obesity is imperative, and weight loss is a key component of this effort. While societal attitudes often emphasize appearance and aesthetics, the true significance of weight loss lies in its potential to enhance health and well-being. Even modest weight loss can lead to significant improvements in metabolic markers, such as blood pressure, blood sugar levels, and cholesterol levels. This, in turn, reduces the risk of obesity-related diseases.

Effective weight loss goes beyond crash diets and extreme measures. A holistic approach considers the underlying factors contributing to weight gain, including genetics, lifestyle, environment, and psychological factors. It involves making sustainable changes to dietary habits, increasing physical activity, managing stress, and cultivating a positive relationship with food.

One of the challenges in addressing obesity is the cycle of weight regain that many individuals experience after initial weight loss. This cycle can be discouraging and lead to feelings of failure. However, understanding the factors that contribute to this cycle—such as hormonal changes and psychological triggers—can help individuals develop strategies to maintain their weight loss over the long term.

The journey to weight loss is not solely about shedding pounds; it's about gaining control over one's health and life. Successful weight loss can boost self-confidence, improve energy levels, and enhance overall quality of life. It allows individuals to engage in activities they might have avoided due to their weight, leading to a more fulfilling and active lifestyle. Moreover, weight loss can increase life expectancy by reducing the risk of obesity-related diseases and complications.

Addressing obesity and pursuing weight loss is a multifaceted endeavor that requires commitment, support, and a positive mindset. It's about acknowledging the impact of excess

weight on both personal well-being and society at large. By adopting a holistic approach to weight loss, individuals can reclaim their health, happiness, and vitality.

In the forthcoming chapters, we will explore strategies for overcoming food cravings, adopting a balanced and nutrient-rich diet, and embracing mindful eating practices. These tools will empower individuals to take charge of their eating habits and work toward a healthier weight, ultimately contributing to a brighter and more vibrant future.

•*Understanding the Battle Against Food Cravings*

Food cravings are a common phenomenon experienced by individuals of all ages and backgrounds. These intense desires for specific foods often strike unexpectedly, leading us to indulge in comfort foods, sugary treats, or savory delights. While the occasional indulgence might seem harmless, persistent and overpowering cravings can contribute to obesity, weight gain, and compromised overall health. In this chapter, we delve deep into the mechanisms behind food cravings, exploring the psychological, physiological, and environmental factors that play a pivotal role in this ongoing battle.

The Psychology of Food Cravings

Food cravings are not solely about hunger and nourishment. They are intricately tied to our emotions, memories, and psychological states. Many people find themselves craving foods that are associated with positive memories or emotions. A scoop of ice cream might remind us of childhood summers, while a slice of pizza could evoke memories of shared laughter with friends. These emotional connections to food create a powerful incentive to give in to cravings.

Moreover, our brains are wired to seek pleasure and avoid discomfort. Certain foods, often high in sugars and fats, activate reward centers in the brain, releasing neurotransmitters like dopamine that generate feelings of pleasure and satisfaction. This positive reinforcement strengthens the link between these foods and the pleasurable sensations they provide, making us more likely to crave them in the future.

Hormones and Physiology

Beyond psychology, hormones and physiological factors also contribute to food cravings. Hormones like ghrelin, known as the "hunger hormone," increase before meals and decrease after eating, influencing appetite and cravings. Leptin, on the other hand, plays a role in satiety and informs the brain when the body is full. Imbalances in these hormones, often caused by irregular eating patterns or inadequate sleep, can amplify cravings.

Stress is another significant factor. When stressed, the body releases cortisol, which can trigger cravings for high-calorie comfort foods. Stress eating is a common coping mechanism, as indulging in certain foods can offer temporary relief from tension. Unfortunately, this can establish a harmful cycle, where stress leads to cravings and overeating, which in turn leads to guilt and more stress.

Environmental Triggers

The environment we inhabit is rich with cues that stimulate cravings. Food advertisements, social media, and even the sights and smells of food while walking down the street can ignite our desire for specific dishes. Additionally, social situations and peer influence can strongly impact our food choices. If everyone around us is indulging, we may feel compelled to join in, regardless of our initial intentions.

The Vicious Cycle

Food cravings can lead to a vicious cycle that poses a significant challenge. Giving in to cravings often provides momentary relief but can lead to feelings of guilt and self-criticism afterward. This emotional turmoil can trigger more cravings as individuals turn to food for comfort.

Breaking this cycle requires understanding and addressing the underlying emotional and physiological triggers.

Empowerment Through Awareness

Understanding the multifaceted nature of food cravings empowers us to take control of our responses. Recognizing that cravings are not solely a matter of willpower allows us to approach them with self-compassion and a strategic mindset. By identifying emotional triggers, acknowledging the influence of hormones, and becoming aware of environmental cues, we can develop effective strategies to manage and eventually overcome persistent cravings.

In the upcoming chapters, we will delve deeper into these strategies, exploring how to differentiate between emotional and physical cravings, building a lifestyle that resists the allure of unhealthy foods, and harnessing the power of mindfulness to regain control over our eating habits. The battle against food cravings is not insurmountable; armed with knowledge and a proactive approach, we can pave the way toward a healthier relationship with food and a more balanced, vibrant life.

Chapter Two

The Science of Cravings

•*Unveiling the Psychology Behind Food Urges*

Food urges, often referred to as cravings, are powerful and irresistible desires for specific types of food. They can strike unexpectedly, leading individuals to seek out and consume certain foods even when they're not physically hungry. While cravings can be triggered by a variety of factors, they are deeply intertwined with the intricate workings of the human mind and psyche. In this chapter, we explore the psychology behind food urges, delving into the emotional, cognitive, and neurological factors that contribute to their emergence and persistence.

Emotional Triggers

Emotions play a central role in the genesis of food urges. People often turn to comfort foods as a way to cope with negative emotions, stress, boredom, or even loneliness. The act of eating certain foods can provide a temporary sense of relief or pleasure, which is why individuals might find themselves reaching for a bar of chocolate after a tough day.

Emotional triggers are not limited to negative feelings; positive emotions can also prompt food cravings. Celebratory events, social gatherings, and joyful occasions are often associated with indulgent foods. The brain forms strong connections between these positive experiences and the foods consumed during them, leading to future cravings when similar emotions arise.

Neurological Reward System

The brain's reward system, primarily governed by the release of neurotransmitters such as dopamine, plays a crucial role in the psychology of food urges. Certain foods, particularly those high in sugars and fats, have the potential to activate the brain's pleasure centers in a way that triggers feelings of enjoyment and satisfaction. This positive reinforcement creates a cycle: consuming these foods leads to pleasurable sensations, which in turn strengthens the desire to seek out and consume them again.

This neurological response is similar to how addictive substances affect the brain. In fact, studies have shown that the brain's response to certain highly palatable foods can mirror the brain's response to drugs of abuse, highlighting the potential addictive nature of certain foods.

Conditioned Responses

The psychology behind food urges is also influenced by classical conditioning. Over time, individuals can develop associations between specific cues and the act of eating certain foods. For example, if someone consistently reaches for potato chips while watching TV, the act of watching TV becomes a trigger for craving potato chips.

These conditioned responses create a link between environmental cues and the urge to eat, even in the absence of hunger. The brain begins to associate certain situations or environments with the reward of eating, leading to cravings when exposed to those cues.

Stress and Cortisol

Stress is a significant driver of food urges. When stress levels rise, the body releases cortisol, a stress hormone. Cortisol can trigger cravings for foods that are high in sugars and fats, as these foods provide a quick source of energy. Additionally, cortisol can influence the brain's reward system, making highly palatable foods even more appealing during times of stress.

Stress eating becomes a coping mechanism for managing emotional discomfort. Consuming these foods might provide temporary relief, but it doesn't address the underlying sources of stress. This cycle can lead to weight gain and increased vulnerability to future stress-induced cravings.

Memory and Food Associations

Memory plays a critical role in the psychology of food urges. People often develop strong associations between certain foods and specific memories or experiences. For instance, the smell of freshly baked cookies might trigger memories of childhood and feelings of warmth and comfort.

These memory associations can lead to cravings for the foods associated with positive memories. The brain seeks to recreate the pleasurable sensations linked to those memories, driving individuals to seek out and consume those foods.

Cognitive Factors

Cognitive factors, including thoughts, beliefs, and attitudes about food, also influence food urges. Dieters, for example, often experience heightened cravings for forbidden foods. The act of labeling certain foods as "off-limits" can paradoxically increase their desirability. The mental battle between the desire to indulge and the effort to adhere to dietary rules can create a psychological strain that intensifies cravings.

Social influences also come into play. Social interactions and peer pressure can shape food choices and cravings. The desire to fit in or to share common experiences with friends and family can lead individuals to consume foods they might not crave otherwise.

The Role of Mindfulness

Mindfulness, the practice of being fully present and nonjudgmental in the moment, can be a powerful tool in managing food urges. Mindfulness helps individuals become more aware of their thoughts, feelings, and bodily sensations, allowing them to recognize cravings without immediately acting on them.

By cultivating mindfulness, individuals can create a space between the emergence of a craving and the decision to act on it. This pause allows for greater self-awareness and the opportunity to make intentional choices rather than giving in to impulsive urges.

The psychology behind food urges is a complex interplay of emotions, memories, brain chemistry, and learned behaviors. Understanding these factors is crucial for managing and overcoming cravings. By recognizing the role of emotions, neurological reward systems, conditioned responses, and cognitive influences, individuals can develop strategies to navigate food urges in a way that aligns with their goals for health and well-being. Mindfulness, emotional awareness, and developing a positive relationship with food are essential tools in unraveling the intricate psychology behind food urges and regaining control over eating behaviors.

•*The Role of Brain Chemistry in Craving Control*

Cravings, those intense and often irresistible desires for specific foods, are intricately tied to the complex workings of the human brain. At the heart of the psychology of cravings lies brain chemistry, a symphony of neurotransmitters, receptors, and neural pathways that govern our thoughts, behaviors, and emotions. Understanding the role of brain chemistry in craving control is key to unraveling the mystery behind why cravings occur and how they can be managed. In this chapter, we delve into the fascinating interplay between brain chemistry and the dynamics of craving control.

Neurotransmitters and Reward Pathways

Central to the role of brain chemistry in cravings is the brain's reward system, which is centered around the release of neurotransmitters—chemical messengers that transmit signals between nerve cells. Dopamine, often referred to as the "feel-good" neurotransmitter, plays a critical role in the experience of pleasure and reward. When we engage in pleasurable activities, such as eating certain foods, dopamine is released in the brain, creating a sense of enjoyment and reinforcing the behavior.

Foods that are high in sugars and fats have a unique ability to stimulate the release of dopamine in the brain. This surge of dopamine contributes to the pleasurable sensations associated with consuming these foods, creating a neurological link between the act of eating and the ensuing feelings of reward.

Hijacking the Reward System

Certain foods, especially those that are highly processed and engineered to be hyper-palatable, have the potential to hijack the brain's reward system. The rapid and intense release of dopamine in response to these foods can lead to a heightened sense of pleasure and satisfaction, making them more desirable. Over time, this can create a cycle of seeking out these foods to replicate the pleasurable experience.

In a sense, the brain chemistry associated with certain foods can lead to a form of addiction. The repeated exposure to highly rewarding foods can alter brain circuitry, leading to a decreased response to dopamine and a reduced sense of reward. This phenomenon, known as "reward deficiency," can drive individuals to consume more of these foods in an attempt to regain the pleasurable sensations they once experienced.

The Influence of Serotonin

Serotonin, another neurotransmitter, also plays a role in the psychology of cravings. Serotonin is often associated with mood regulation and feelings of well-being. Low levels of serotonin have been linked to increased impulsivity and a propensity for emotional eating.

Consuming certain foods, particularly those high in carbohydrates, can temporarily boost serotonin levels and create a sense of calm and contentment. This might explain why individuals often crave carbohydrate-rich comfort foods during times of stress or emotional turmoil.

Hormonal Regulation of Appetite

Brain chemistry also extends to the hormonal regulation of appetite. Hormones like ghrelin, known as the "hunger hormone," and leptin, known as the "satiety hormone," play crucial roles in appetite and cravings.

Ghrelin signals hunger and prompts individuals to seek out food. It increases before meals and decreases after eating. Ghrelin levels are influenced by factors such as sleep patterns, stress, and meal timing. Disruptions in ghrelin regulation can lead to increased cravings, especially for calorie-dense foods.

Leptin, on the other hand, informs the brain when the body is satiated. Leptin levels rise as fat stores increase, signaling to the brain that it's time to stop eating. However, individuals with obesity often develop resistance to leptin, leading to a diminished response to its signals of fullness. This resistance can perpetuate overeating and cravings.

Stress and the HPA Axis

Stress, a powerful trigger for cravings, involves the interaction of the hypothalamus-pituitary-adrenal (HPA) axis. In response to stress, the hypothalamus releases corticotropin-releasing hormone (CRH), which signals the pituitary gland to release adrenocorticotropic hormone (ACTH). ACTH then stimulates the adrenal glands to produce cortisol, a stress hormone.

Cortisol, in turn, influences brain chemistry and cravings. It can stimulate the brain's reward system and lead to cravings for high-calorie, pleasurable foods. Additionally, cortisol can affect blood sugar levels, increasing the desire for quick sources of energy, often found in sugary foods.

The Gut-Brain Connection

The gut, often referred to as the "second brain," also plays a role in the psychology of cravings. The gut is home to a complex network of neurons and neurotransmitters that communicate with the brain. This gut-brain connection, known as the gut-brain axis, influences appetite, mood, and even cravings.

The gut microbiota, the diverse community of microorganisms residing in the digestive tract, can impact brain chemistry and cravings. Certain bacteria in the gut are involved in the fermentation of dietary fibers, producing short-chain fatty acids that influence the release of neurotransmitters. Changes in the gut microbiota composition have been linked to alterations in brain function and behavior, including cravings.

Regaining Control

Understanding the intricate role of brain chemistry in cravings is a crucial step toward regaining control over eating behaviors. While brain chemistry can drive the emergence and persistence of cravings, it's not a deterministic factor. The brain is adaptable and can be rewired through intentional choices and behavioral changes.

Mindfulness, for example, can help individuals become more aware of the neurological responses driving cravings. By observing cravings without immediate reactivity, individuals can create a space to make conscious choices rather than succumbing to impulsive urges.

Adopting a balanced and nutrient-rich diet can also influence brain chemistry. Nutrients like omega-3 fatty acids and antioxidants found in fruits, vegetables, and fatty fish can support brain health and balance neurotransmitter production.

The role of brain chemistry in craving control is a dynamic and intricate interplay between neurotransmitters, hormones, neural pathways, and gut-brain interactions. While certain foods have the ability to hijack the brain's reward system and create addictive-like responses, understanding these mechanisms empowers individuals to make informed choices.

By cultivating awareness, mindfulness, and a deep understanding of the brain's response to certain foods, individuals can develop strategies to manage cravings and create a healthier relationship with food. The journey toward craving control involves harnessing the power of brain chemistry to align eating behaviors with one's health and well-being goals.

Chapter Three
Mapping Your Cravings

•Identifying Trigger Foods and Situations

The quest for healthier eating often begins with the recognition that certain foods and situations have the power to trigger intense cravings and overeating. These trigger foods and situations can undermine efforts to maintain a balanced diet and make it challenging to achieve health and wellness goals. In this chapter, we delve into the art of identifying trigger foods and situations, exploring the psychological, physiological, and environmental factors that contribute to their influence, and discussing strategies to regain control and make informed choices.

Understanding Trigger Foods

Trigger foods are those that evoke powerful cravings and compulsive eating behaviors. These foods often have a specific combination of taste, texture, and sensory appeal that create an intense desire to consume them. Trigger foods can vary widely from person to person, but they tend to share some common characteristics.

Highly processed and hyper-palatable foods are often trigger foods. These foods are engineered to maximize taste and pleasure, containing combinations of sugars, unhealthy fats, and additives that stimulate the brain's reward centers. The rapid release of dopamine in response to these foods creates a sense of pleasure and satisfaction, reinforcing the desire to consume them.

Identifying Your Trigger Foods

Identifying your personal trigger foods requires self-awareness and introspection. Start by keeping a food journal to track your eating habits and the emotions or situations that accompany them. Take note of instances when you find yourself craving specific foods intensely. Reflect on whether these cravings are linked to certain emotions, times of day, or external cues.

It's important to differentiate between true physiological hunger and emotional cravings. Emotional cravings often arise suddenly, with a specific desire for a particular food. Physiological hunger, on the other hand, tends to build gradually and can be satisfied with a variety of nutrient-rich options.

Emotional Triggers

Emotional triggers play a significant role in the identification of trigger foods. Emotions such as stress, boredom, loneliness, sadness, and anxiety can lead to cravings for comfort foods. These foods provide a sense of temporary relief from uncomfortable emotions, but they do not address the underlying issues.

Take note of how your emotional state affects your food choices. If you find yourself consistently turning to specific foods during times of emotional distress, those foods may be your trigger foods. Developing alternative coping mechanisms, such as deep breathing, exercise, or talking to a friend, can help break the cycle of emotional eating.

Social and Environmental Triggers

Social situations and environmental cues can also trigger cravings. Being in the presence of certain foods, such as at parties or gatherings, can prompt a desire to indulge. Peer pressure, the availability of specific foods, and the influence of others' eating behaviors can all contribute to cravings for trigger foods.

Pay attention to situations where you're more likely to encounter your trigger foods. Make a conscious effort to plan ahead and have healthier alternatives available in those situations. Communicate your dietary preferences and goals to friends and family to gain their support and understanding.

The Role of Portion Sizes

Portion sizes can also act as triggers. For some individuals, starting to eat a trigger food can trigger a strong desire to finish the entire portion, even if they were not initially hungry. The "all-or-nothing" mentality can be challenging to overcome.

Experiment with portion control techniques, such as using smaller plates, serving yourself a predetermined amount, and practicing mindful eating. Mindful eating involves savoring each bite, paying attention to the taste, texture, and satisfaction that each mouthful provides.

Physical Cues

Physical cues, such as changes in energy levels, can indicate the presence of cravings. When blood sugar levels drop, it can trigger cravings for quick sources of energy, often found in sugary foods. Lack of sleep and dehydration can also amplify cravings for unhealthy foods.

Prioritize balanced meals that include a combination of protein, healthy fats, and fiber-rich carbohydrates. Eating at regular intervals and staying hydrated can help stabilize blood sugar levels and reduce the likelihood of sudden cravings.

Creating a Trigger Foods List

Creating a trigger foods list can be a helpful tool in your journey to identifying and managing triggers. Write down the foods that consistently evoke cravings or lead to overeating. Be honest with yourself about which foods have a strong hold over your eating behaviors.

Once you've identified your trigger foods, you can develop strategies to minimize their influence. This might involve gradually reducing your consumption of these foods, finding healthier alternatives, and reframing your mindset about these foods. Keep in mind that avoiding trigger foods entirely may not always be necessary or sustainable; instead, focus on building a healthier relationship with them.

Strategies for Craving Control

Once you've identified your trigger foods and situations, you can implement various strategies to regain control over your eating behaviors:

1. Mindfulness: Develop mindfulness around your eating habits. Pay attention to your thoughts, emotions, and physical sensations before, during, and after eating. This awareness can help you distinguish between true hunger and emotional cravings.
2. Emotional Regulation: Practice healthy ways of managing emotions that do not involve turning to food for comfort. Engage in activities you enjoy, practice relaxation techniques, or seek support from friends, family, or professionals.
3. Substitution: Identify healthier alternatives to your trigger foods. Experiment with nutritious options that provide similar flavors and textures without triggering intense cravings.
4. Preparation: Plan ahead for situations where you're likely to encounter trigger foods. Have a strategy in place, such as eating a balanced meal before attending an event or bringing your own healthier snacks.
5. Portion Control: Practice portion control by using smaller plates and serving sizes. Focus on savoring each bite and listening to your body's signals of fullness.
6. Food Environment: Create an environment that supports your goals. Keep trigger foods out of sight and stock your pantry with nutrient-rich options that are aligned with your dietary preferences.
7. Distraction: Engage in activities that shift your focus away from cravings. Take a walk, read a book, or engage in a hobby that brings you joy.
8. Support System: Share your goals and challenges with a supportive friend, family member, or accountability partner. Having someone to lean on can make a significant difference in managing trigger foods.
9. Seek Professional Guidance: If trigger foods are significantly impacting your well-being, consider seeking guidance from a registered dietitian, therapist, or healthcare professional who specializes in emotional eating and cravings.

Identifying trigger foods and situations is a crucial step in the journey toward healthier eating habits. By becoming aware of the psychological, physiological, and environmental factors that contribute to cravings, individuals can develop strategies to regain control over their eating behaviors. The process involves cultivating self-awareness, practicing mindfulness, and building a toolbox of techniques to manage cravings and make informed choices aligned with health and well-being goals.

•*Recognizing Emotional vs. Physical Cravings*

Cravings are a universal experience, often accompanied by a strong desire to indulge in specific foods. However, not all cravings are created equal. There's a crucial distinction between emotional cravings and physical hunger, and recognizing this difference is key to making mindful and health-conscious eating choices. In this chapter, we explore the nuances of emotional and physical cravings, shedding light on their origins, characteristics, and strategies to differentiate and manage them effectively.

Emotional cravings, also known as psychological cravings, are cravings driven by emotions rather than physiological hunger. These cravings are often tied to specific feelings, such as stress, boredom, sadness, or anxiety. The desire to consume certain foods arises as a means of seeking comfort, pleasure, or distraction from these emotions.

Characteristics of Emotional Cravings

Emotional cravings are characterized by several distinct features:

1. Sudden Onset: Emotional cravings can arise suddenly and intensify rapidly. You may find yourself fixated on a specific food, feeling compelled to consume it immediately.
2. Specific Food Choice: Emotional cravings are often tied to specific foods with strong sensory appeal, such as chocolate, ice cream, or chips. The desire is not merely to satisfy hunger but to experience the taste and texture of a particular food.
3. Lack of Physical Hunger: One of the key differentiators of emotional cravings is the absence of true physical hunger. Even if you've recently eaten a substantial meal, you may still experience a powerful desire for a specific food.
4. Emotional Triggers: Emotional cravings are closely linked to emotions and situations. Stressful days, feeling lonely, or dealing with challenging emotions can trigger a strong desire for comfort foods.

Origins of Emotional Cravings

Emotional cravings are rooted in the complex interplay between emotions and brain chemistry. Stress, for instance, can lead to the release of cortisol, a stress hormone that influences food preferences. The brain's reward system, particularly the release of dopamine, also comes into play. Comfort foods often trigger a release of dopamine, creating a temporary sense of pleasure and relief from emotional distress.

Managing Emotional Cravings

Recognizing and managing emotional cravings is crucial for maintaining a healthy relationship with food and preventing overeating. Here are strategies to help manage emotional cravings:

1. Practice Mindfulness: Develop mindfulness around your emotions and cravings. Pause and ask yourself whether you're truly hungry or if you're seeking comfort or distraction from emotions.
2. Emotional Awareness: Identify the emotions that trigger your cravings. Keep a journal to track your emotions and the foods you crave. This awareness can help you establish patterns and develop alternative coping strategies.
3. Coping Mechanisms: Explore healthy ways to manage emotions without turning to food. Engage in activities you enjoy, practice deep breathing, meditate, or connect with friends and family for support.
4. Delay Gratification: When an emotional craving arises, commit to waiting for a set period before indulging. During this time, engage in an activity to distract yourself and assess whether the craving subsides.
5. Substitution: If you recognize that an emotional craving is not tied to true hunger, consider substituting the desired food with a healthier alternative that still satisfies your senses.

Defining Physical Hunger

Physical hunger, also known as biological hunger, is the body's natural response to a need for sustenance. It's a physiological signal that the body requires nutrients and energy to function optimally.

Physical hunger is an essential bodily sensation that signals the need for nourishment. When you experience physical hunger, your body sends signals to your brain, such as stomach growling or a feeling of emptiness. It's important to listen to your body's hunger cues and provide it with the nutrients it needs through balanced meals and snacks. Ignoring physical hunger can lead to low energy levels, difficulty concentrating, and potential overeating later on. Remember to fuel your body with healthy and satisfying foods when you feel physically hungry.

Characteristics of Physical Hunger

Physical hunger displays several distinct characteristics:

1. Gradual Build-up: Physical hunger builds gradually over time. You may notice increasing stomach rumbling, a sensation of emptiness, or a decline in energy levels.
2. General Food Craving: Unlike emotional cravings that focus on specific foods, physical hunger is usually accompanied by a general desire for a variety of foods.
3. Satiety with Food: True physical hunger is satisfied by eating a balanced meal. You'll likely experience a sense of fullness and satisfaction after consuming a reasonable portion.
4. Absence of Emotional Triggers: Physical hunger isn't linked to emotions or external triggers. It's a natural response to the body's need for nourishment.

Origins of Physical Hunger

Physical hunger is regulated by various hormones and biological signals. The hormone ghrelin, often referred to as the "hunger hormone," increases before meals and decreases after eating. Ghrelin levels rise when the stomach is empty, sending signals to the brain that it's time to eat.

Blood sugar levels also play a role in triggering physical hunger. As blood sugar levels drop, the body signals hunger to replenish energy stores.

Managing Physical Hunger

Recognizing physical hunger is essential for providing your body with the nourishment it needs. Here are strategies to help manage physical hunger:

1. Eat Regularly: Honor your body's hunger signals by eating regular meals and snacks. Consistent eating patterns help stabilize blood sugar levels and prevent extreme hunger.
2. Balanced Meals: Consume balanced meals that include a variety of nutrients. Protein, healthy fats, and fiber-rich carbohydrates can provide sustained energy and promote satiety.
3. Mindful Eating: Practice mindful eating by paying attention to your body's hunger and fullness cues. Eat slowly and savor each bite to fully experience the satisfaction of a meal.
4. Stay Hydrated: Sometimes, feelings of hunger can be mistaken for dehydration. Drink water throughout the day to ensure you're properly hydrated.

Differentiating and Managing Cravings

Differentiating between emotional cravings and physical hunger is an ongoing practice that involves self-awareness and a deeper understanding of your body's signals. Here are strategies to help you differentiate and manage cravings effectively:

1. Pause and Reflect: Before reaching for a particular food, pause and reflect on whether you're experiencing true hunger or an emotional craving. Consider whether you've eaten recently and whether your body is signaling physical signs of hunger.
2. Label Your Cravings: When a craving arises, label it as either an emotional craving or a sign of physical hunger. This simple act of labeling can help you gain perspective and respond intentionally.
3. Check In with Emotions: Tune into your emotional state. If you're feeling stressed, sad, anxious, or bored, there's a higher likelihood that the craving is emotional. Consider alternative ways to address these emotions without turning to food.
4. Time Delay: When a craving strikes, practice delaying your response. Engage in a different activity, such as taking a short walk or engaging in a hobby, to create a space between the craving and your response.
5. Choose Nutrient-Rich Foods: If you're genuinely hungry, opt for nutrient-rich, whole foods that provide sustained energy and satiety. Prioritize foods that nourish your body and align with your health goals.
6. Seek Support: If you find that emotional cravings are a recurring challenge, consider seeking support from a therapist, counselor, or support group. Addressing underlying emotional triggers can have a positive impact on your relationship with food.
7. Practice Self-Compassion: Be kind to yourself throughout this process. Recognize that managing cravings is a skill that takes time to develop. If you do give in to a craving, avoid self-judgment and focus on moving forward.

Recognizing emotional cravings versus physical hunger is a journey that requires self-awareness, mindfulness, and a willingness to listen to your body's signals. By understanding the origins, characteristics, and implications of both types of cravings, you can make more informed and intentional choices about the foods you consume. Cultivating a deeper connection with your body's needs and emotions empowers you to respond to cravings in ways that support your overall health and well-being.

Chapter Four

Building a Craving-Resistant Lifestyle

•*Crafting a Balanced and Nutrient-Rich D*Die

The pursuit of optimal health and well-being begins with the foundation of a balanced and nutrient-rich diet. A diet that provides a variety of essential nutrients in the right proportions can support physical and mental vitality, boost immunity, and reduce the risk of chronic diseases. Crafting such a diet involves making informed choices about the types of foods you consume and the way you structure your meals. In this chapter, we explore the principles of creating a balanced and nutrient-rich diet, from understanding macronutrients and micronutrients to practical tips for meal planning and mindful eating.

Understanding Macronutrients and Micronutrients

Macronutrients and micronutrients are two categories of essential nutrients that the body requires for optimal function.

Macronutrients:

1. Carbohydrates: Carbohydrates are the body's primary source of energy. Complex carbohydrates, found in whole grains, fruits, vegetables, and legumes, provide sustained energy and fiber. Simple carbohydrates, such as sugars and refined grains, offer quick bursts of energy but lack essential nutrients.

2. Proteins: Proteins are crucial for building and repairing tissues, producing enzymes and hormones, and supporting immune function. Sources of high-quality protein include lean meats, poultry, fish, eggs, dairy products, legumes, nuts, and seeds.

3. Fats: Healthy fats are essential for cell structure, hormone production, and absorbing fat-soluble vitamins. Unsaturated fats, found in foods like avocados, nuts, seeds, and olive oil, are beneficial for heart health. Limit saturated and trans fats found in processed and fried foods.

Micronutrients:

1. Vitamins: Vitamins are essential for various bodily functions, such as metabolism, immune response, and bone health. Sources include fruits, vegetables, whole grains, lean proteins, and dairy products.

2. Minerals: Minerals play a role in bone health, fluid balance, nerve function, and energy production. Calcium, magnesium, iron, zinc, and potassium are examples of important minerals found in a variety of foods.

Building a Balanced Plate

Creating a balanced plate involves including a variety of foods from each food group to ensure you're getting all the necessary nutrients.

1. Half Your Plate with Vegetables and Fruits: Vegetables and fruits are rich in vitamins, minerals, fiber, and antioxidants. Aim to fill half of your plate with a colorful array of these nutrient-packed foods.

2. Quarter with Lean Proteins: Include a lean protein source, such as lean meats, poultry, fish, eggs, legumes, or tofu, to support muscle health and provide essential amino acids.

3. Quarter with Whole Grains or Starchy Vegetables:** Choose whole grains like quinoa, brown rice, whole wheat pasta, and whole-grain bread to provide complex carbohydrates and fiber. Starchy vegetables like sweet potatoes and corn also provide healthy carbohydrates.

4. Incorporate Healthy Fats: Include sources of healthy fats, such as avocados, nuts, seeds, and olive oil, to support brain health, hormone production, and nutrient absorption.

5. Dairy or Dairy Alternatives: Dairy products or fortified dairy alternatives provide calcium, vitamin D, and protein. Opt for low-fat or fat-free options to limit saturated fat intake.

Strategies for Nutrient-Rich Eating

Crafting a nutrient-rich diet goes beyond individual meals; it involves making consistent choices that prioritize your health. Here are strategies to help you achieve a nutrient-rich eating pattern:

1. Eat a Rainbow of Colors: Different colors in fruits and vegetables indicate a variety of vitamins, minerals, and antioxidants. Aim to consume a wide range of colors to ensure you're getting a diverse array of nutrients.

2. Prioritize Whole Foods: Choose whole, minimally processed foods over highly processed options. Whole foods retain more nutrients and are often higher in fiber and antioxidants.

3. Read Labels: When purchasing packaged foods, read labels to understand their nutritional content. Look for foods with fewer added sugars, sodium, and unhealthy fats.

4. Mindful Portions: Practice portion control to prevent overeating. Focus on intuitive eating by tuning in to your body's hunger and fullness cues.

5. Variety is Key: Include a variety of foods from different food groups to ensure you're getting a broad spectrum of nutrients. Experiment with new foods and recipes to keep meals exciting.

6. Hydration: Drink plenty of water throughout the day to stay hydrated and support various bodily functions.

Meal Planning for Nutrient-Rich Eating

Meal planning can play a significant role in maintaining a nutrient-rich diet. Here's how to create well-rounded meals:

1. Plan Balanced Meals: When planning meals, aim to include a source of lean protein, a variety of vegetables, a complex carbohydrate, and a source of healthy fats.

2. Batch Cooking: Prepare larger quantities of staple ingredients like grains, proteins, and roasted vegetables to use throughout the week. This saves time and helps you avoid relying on less nutritious convenience foods.

3. Pack in Nutrient-Dense Snacks: Keep nutrient-rich snacks, such as cut-up vegetables, fruits, nuts, and yogurt, readily available for when hunger strikes between meals.

4. Incorporate Plant-Based Proteins: Include plant-based protein sources like beans, lentils, quinoa, and tofu to increase variety and reduce reliance on animal products.

5. Plan for Color: Aim to include a variety of colorful fruits and vegetables in each meal to ensure you're getting a diverse range of nutrients.

6. Mindful Eating: Practice mindful eating by savoring each bite, eating slowly, and paying attention to how your body responds to different foods.

Common Nutrient Deficiencies and Prevention

Certain nutrients are more likely to be deficient in specific diets or populations. Taking steps to address potential deficiencies can support overall health:

1. Vitamin D: Vitamin D deficiency is common, especially in regions with limited sunlight. Include vitamin D-rich foods like fatty fish, egg yolks, fortified dairy products, and spend time outdoors.

2. Iron: Iron deficiency is prevalent, particularly among menstruating women and vegetarians. Include iron-rich foods like lean meats, poultry, fish, beans, lentils, and fortified cereals. Pair plant-based iron sources with vitamin C-rich foods to enhance absorption.

3. Calcium: Calcium is essential for bone health. Include dairy products, fortified dairy alternatives, leafy greens, almonds, and chia seeds to meet your calcium needs.

4. Omega-3 Fatty Acids: Omega-3 fatty acids are important for heart health and brain function. Include fatty fish (salmon, mackerel, sardines), flaxseeds, chia seeds, and walnuts.

5. B Vitamins: B vitamins play a role in energy production and metabolism. Include a variety of whole grains, lean proteins, and leafy greens to ensure you're getting a range of B vitamins.

Crafting a balanced and nutrient-rich diet is a journey that involves making informed choices about the foods you consume and the way you structure your meals. By understanding macronutrients, micronutrients, and the principles of balanced eating, you can create meals that support your health and well-being. Prioritizing whole, minimally processed foods, incorporating a variety of colors and nutrient sources, and practicing mindful eating all contribute to nourishing your body and promoting optimal health. Remember that small, consistent steps toward nutrient-rich eating can have a profound impact on your overall well-being over time.

•*Incorporating Mindful Eating Practices*

In a world characterized by busy schedules, distractions, and on-the-go eating, the concept of mindful eating offers a refreshing and transformative approach to nourishing our bodies and minds. Mindful eating encourages us to slow down, be present, and savor every bite, fostering a deeper connection with the food we consume. This practice not only enhances our enjoyment of meals but also promotes a healthier relationship with food, improved digestion, and a greater sense of overall well-being. In this chapter, we explore the principles and benefits of mindful eating and provide practical strategies for incorporating this practice into your daily life.

Mindful eating is rooted in mindfulness, a practice that involves being fully present and engaged in the current moment without judgment. Mindful eating extends this concept to the realm of food and nourishment, inviting us to pay attention to the sensory experience of eating, including taste, smell, texture, and the act of chewing.

Principles of Mindful Eating

1. Awareness: Mindful eating begins with cultivating awareness. This involves noticing the physical sensations of hunger and fullness, becoming attuned to the flavors and textures of the food, and recognizing emotional and environmental cues that influence eating.

2. Non-Judgment: Mindful eating is free from judgment or criticism. It involves observing your thoughts and feelings without labeling them as "good" or "bad." This non-judgmental awareness fosters a compassionate approach to yourself and your eating habits.
3. Savoring: Savoring each bite involves fully experiencing the tastes and textures of the food. Taking your time to chew slowly and appreciate the flavors contributes to a heightened sense of satisfaction and enjoyment.
4. Presence: Being fully present during meals means minimizing distractions and giving your full attention to the act of eating. Put away electronic devices, turn off the TV, and create a calm and inviting eating environment.

Benefits of Mindful Eating

Practicing mindful eating offers a range of physical, mental, and emotional benefits:

1. Improved Digestion: Mindful eating promotes proper digestion by allowing the body to focus on the process of chewing, breaking down food, and releasing digestive enzymes.
2. Enhanced Satiety: By paying attention to hunger and fullness cues, you're more likely to eat until you're satisfied, rather than overeating. This supports weight management and prevents discomfort from overconsumption.
3. Emotional Regulation: Mindful eating helps you become more attuned to emotional triggers that influence eating. This awareness allows you to choose alternative coping mechanisms for stress, boredom, or sadness.
4. Reduced Binge Eating: By practicing non-judgmental awareness, you can identify patterns of binge eating and address the emotional roots that contribute to this behavior.
5. Body Awareness: Mindful eating encourages body awareness, helping you develop a more compassionate relationship with your body and its needs.
6. Enjoyment of Food: Savoring each bite leads to a greater appreciation for the tastes, textures, and aromas of food, enhancing the overall eating experience.

Incorporating Mindful Eating Practices

Incorporating mindful eating into your routine requires intention, practice, and patience. Here are practical strategies to help you cultivate this transformative practice:

1. Start Small: Begin by choosing one meal or snack each day to practice mindful eating. As you become more comfortable, gradually expand the practice to other meals.
2. Create a Calm Environment: Choose a quiet, comfortable space to enjoy your meals. Set the table, dim the lights, and eliminate distractions.
3. Engage Your Senses: Before taking a bite, take a moment to observe the colors, textures, and aromas of your food. Notice any sensations of anticipation or desire.
4. Chew Slowly: Chew each bite slowly and deliberately. Pay attention to the flavors that emerge as you chew.

5. Put Down Utensils: Put down your fork or spoon between bites. This encourages a pace that allows you to fully experience and savor the food.
6. Check In with Hunger and Fullness: Pause during your meal to check in with your hunger and fullness levels. Notice the gradual shift from hunger to satisfaction.
7. Practice the 5 S's: As you eat, engage with the "Five S's" of mindful eating: Savor, Swallow, Set down utensils, Sit back, and Smile.
8. Limit Distractions: Turn off screens, put away your phone, and engage in conversation or silent reflection as you eat.
9. Mindful Snacking: Apply mindful eating to snacks as well. Choose nutrient-rich snacks and take time to savor each bite.
10. Observe Emotions: Notice any emotions that arise during the meal. If you find yourself turning to food for emotional comfort, acknowledge it without judgment.
11. Practice Gratitude: Before you start eating, take a moment to express gratitude for the nourishment in front of you. This shifts your mindset and enhances your connection to the food.

Applying Mindful Eating Beyond Meals

Mindful eating doesn't need to be limited to formal meal times. You can apply these principles to various eating experiences throughout your day:

1. Eating on the Go: Even when eating on the go, take a moment to pause, breathe, and engage with your food. Mindful eating is possible regardless of your surroundings.
2. Mindful Cooking: Approach cooking with the same sense of mindfulness. Pay attention to the ingredients, the smells, and the textures as you prepare your meals.

3. Mindful Grocery Shopping: Practice mindfulness while grocery shopping by observing the colors, textures, and smells of the produce. Plan your meals and snacks mindfully, choosing nutrient-rich options.
4. Eating in Social Settings: Mindful eating can enhance social eating experiences. Engage in conversation, savor the flavors, and appreciate the company of others.

Overcoming Challenges

Incorporating mindful eating may come with challenges, especially if you're used to eating quickly or are easily distracted. Here's how to overcome common obstacles:

1. Impatience: If you're accustomed to eating quickly, remind yourself that this practice is about creating a healthier relationship with food. Allow yourself to slow down and enjoy the experience.
2. Distractions: Turn off electronic devices and find a quiet space to eat. If eating with others, engage in mindful conversation that enhances the meal.

3. Mind Wandering: If your mind wanders, gently bring your attention back to the sensations of eating. Be patient with yourself; the practice improves over time.

Incorporating mindful eating practices offers a transformative approach to nourishing your body and cultivating a healthier relationship with food. By engaging all your senses, savoring each bite, and creating a calm eating environment, you can experience the joy of eating in a more conscious and present way. The benefits of mindful eating extend beyond the plate, enriching your overall well-being and fostering a deeper appreciation for the nourishment that food provides. As you continue to practice, you'll find that mindful eating becomes a valuable tool for making more intentional and health-promoting choices in all aspects of your life.

Chapter Five

Strategies for Craving Management

•Practical Techniques to Curb Sudden Cravings

Sudden cravings for certain foods can feel overwhelming and challenging to resist, especially when they strike unexpectedly. These cravings often seem to come out of nowhere and can be triggered by emotions, environmental cues, or even physiological factors. While it's normal to experience cravings from time to time, finding effective ways to manage them is essential for maintaining a balanced and health-conscious diet. In this chapter, we explore practical techniques to curb sudden cravings, empowering you to make mindful and informed choices when faced with intense desires for specific foods.

1. Pause and Reflect

When a sudden craving hits, take a moment to pause and reflect. Instead of giving in to the craving immediately, give yourself a brief window to consider your options. Ask yourself if you're truly hungry or if the craving is driven by other factors like emotions or stress. This moment of pause allows you to bring awareness to the situation and make a more intentional decision about whether to indulge the craving or choose a healthier alternative.

2. Stay Hydrated

Dehydration can sometimes masquerade as hunger or cravings. When you feel a sudden urge for a specific food, try drinking a glass of water first. Give your body a chance to signal whether the craving was actually related to thirst. Staying hydrated throughout the day can help prevent unnecessary cravings and support overall well-being.

3. Practice Mindfulness

Mindfulness can be a powerful tool for managing sudden cravings. Instead of giving in to the impulse immediately, practice being fully present in the moment. Observe the craving without judgment, and notice any physical sensations, emotions, or thoughts that arise. Mindful awareness can create a space between the craving and your response, allowing you to make a conscious choice about how to proceed.

4. Distract Yourself

Distraction techniques can redirect your focus away from the craving and give it time to subside. Engage in an activity that occupies your mind and hands, such as taking a short walk, doing a puzzle, or engaging in a hobby you enjoy. By the time you're finished, the intensity of the craving may have diminished.

5. Delay Gratification

The "delayed gratification" technique involves agreeing to wait a certain amount of time before indulging in the craving. Set a timer for 10-15 minutes and use that time to engage in a different activity. During this period, reflect on whether the craving is still as strong or if it has diminished. This practice allows you to take control over impulsive decisions and make a more mindful choice.

6. Choose a Healthier Alternative

If you're craving a specific type of food, consider choosing a healthier alternative that still satisfies the craving. For example, if you're craving something sweet, opt for a piece of fruit. If you're craving something crunchy and salty, reach for a small portion of nuts or seeds. Finding nutrient-rich substitutes can help satisfy the craving while supporting your health goals.

7. Practice Portion Control

If the craving persists and you decide to indulge, practice portion control. Instead of consuming an entire portion, serve yourself a small amount and savor each bite mindfully. Pay attention to the taste, texture, and satisfaction that the food provides. This approach allows you to enjoy the food without overindulging.

8. Plan for Occasional Treats

Allowing yourself occasional treats can actually help prevent feelings of deprivation and reduce the intensity of cravings. Plan in advance to enjoy your favorite indulgent foods in moderation. When you know you have the opportunity to enjoy a treat, you may find that the sudden cravings for those foods become less frequent and less intense.

9. Address Underlying Emotions

Sudden cravings can often be linked to underlying emotions or stress. Take a moment to explore whether there's an emotional trigger for the craving. Are you feeling anxious, bored, or stressed? If so, consider addressing the underlying emotion through healthy coping mechanisms like exercise, deep breathing, or engaging in a relaxing activity.

10. Create a Craving Journal

Keeping a craving journal can help you identify patterns and triggers. When a sudden craving arises, jot down the time, the food you're craving, your emotional state, and any other relevant factors. Over time, you may notice trends that provide insight into the circumstances that trigger your cravings. This awareness can help you proactively address those triggers.

11. Practice Gentle Self-Compassion

It's important to approach the management of cravings with a sense of self-compassion. Instead of berating yourself for experiencing a craving, remind yourself that cravings are a natural part of being human. Treat yourself with kindness and understanding as you navigate these moments, and remember that occasional indulgences are normal and can be enjoyed in moderation.

12. Seek Support

If you find that sudden cravings are frequently derailing your health goals, consider seeking support. A registered dietitian or nutritionist can provide personalized strategies for managing cravings and creating a sustainable eating plan that aligns with your preferences and goals. Additionally, connecting with a supportive friend, family member, or accountability partner can provide encouragement and motivation.

Sudden cravings are a common experience, but they don't have to control your eating choices. By implementing practical techniques to curb these cravings, you can make more mindful and intentional decisions about the foods you consume. Whether it's pausing to reflect, staying hydrated, practicing mindfulness, or finding healthier alternatives, these strategies empower you to take control over your eating behaviors and cultivate a balanced and health-conscious approach to your diet. Remember that progress takes time, and each small choice you make in the direction of mindful eating contributes to your overall well-being.

•*Creating a Supportive Environment for Success*

Managing cravings and maintaining a balanced approach to eating requires more than just willpower. The environment in which we live, work, and socialize plays a significant role in shaping our behaviors and choices, including how we respond to cravings. Creating a supportive environment that aligns with your health and wellness goals can be a powerful strategy for successful craving control. In this chapter, we delve into the impact of our surroundings on cravings, explore ways to modify your environment to encourage healthier choices, and provide practical tips for building a conducive atmosphere that supports your journey toward mindful and health-conscious eating.

Our environment encompasses both physical and psychological factors that influence our behaviors and decisions. When it comes to cravings and eating habits, the environment can trigger cues, associations, and triggers that lead to indulgence. Recognizing the role of environment in shaping our choices empowers us to take intentional steps to create a setting that supports our craving control efforts.

Physical Environment:

1. Accessibility: The availability and accessibility of certain foods can significantly impact whether you give in to cravings. If unhealthy snacks and treats are prominently displayed or easily reachable, you're more likely to consume them when cravings strike.
2. Visibility: Foods that are in plain sight are more likely to catch your attention and trigger cravings. Keeping nutrient-rich foods visible can encourage you to make healthier choices.
3. Social Influence: Social situations and peer pressure can shape your eating behaviors. If those around you are indulging in unhealthy foods, you might feel more compelled to join in.
4. Food Placement: Placing healthier options at eye level and less healthy options out of immediate sight can influence your choices. Making nutritious choices the default option can facilitate better eating decisions.

Psychological Environment:

1. Emotional Triggers: Emotional states like stress, boredom, or sadness can trigger cravings. Your environment can influence these emotions. Creating a calming and supportive space can help mitigate emotional triggers.
2. Cues and Associations: Environmental cues, such as the smell of freshly baked goods or the sight of a favorite restaurant, can trigger cravings. Recognizing these cues and finding ways to manage them is essential for successful craving control.
3. Mindset: Your mindset and beliefs about food and cravings are influenced by your environment. Surrounding yourself with positive messaging and reminders of your health goals can reinforce your commitment to mindful eating.

Modifying Your Environment for Success

Creating a supportive environment involves intentional changes to both your physical and psychological surroundings. Here's how to modify your environment to facilitate better craving control:

1. Stock Your Kitchen Thoughtfully:

- Nutrient-Rich Foods: Fill your pantry, refrigerator, and countertops with nutrient-rich foods like fruits, vegetables, lean proteins, whole grains, and healthy fats.
- Pre-Portioned Snacks: If you keep snacks on hand, portion them out into individual servings to avoid overindulging.
- Hide Temptations: If you have foods that trigger cravings, store them out of sight or in less accessible places.

2. Plan Your Meals and Snacks:

- Meal Prep: Prepare balanced meals and snacks in advance to prevent impulsive choices when hunger strikes.
- Mindful Snacking: Keep nutritious snacks on hand, like cut-up vegetables, fruit, nuts, and yogurt, to satisfy hunger and cravings between meals.

3. Create a Mindful Eating Space:

- Designate a Calm Space: Choose a designated area for eating that is free from distractions and conducive to mindful eating.
- Set the Ambiance: Create a calming atmosphere with soft lighting, pleasant music, and comfortable seating.

4. Manage Emotional Triggers:

- Stress Reduction: Create a space for relaxation and stress reduction. Incorporate practices like meditation, deep breathing, or journaling into your daily routine.
- Healthy Coping Mechanisms: Surround yourself with tools and activities that help you manage emotions without turning to food, such as exercise equipment, art supplies, or soothing teas.

5. Surround Yourself with Positive Reminders:

- Visual Cues: Place visual reminders of your health goals in prominent places. This could be a motivational quote, a vision board, or a picture of a role model.
- Mindful Eating Affirmations: Develop a set of mindful eating affirmations and display them where you can see them. These affirmations can remind you of your commitment to health-conscious choices.

6. Engage Social Support:

- Accountability Partners: Share your health goals with friends or family members who can provide encouragement and hold you accountable.
- Healthy Social Outings: Choose restaurants or activities that align with your health goals when socializing. Your environment during social events can impact your choices.

Practical Tips for Creating a Supportive Environment

1. Meal Planning: Invest time in planning your meals and snacks for the week. Having a clear plan reduces the likelihood of succumbing to sudden cravings.
2. Grocery Shopping: Make a shopping list that prioritizes nutrient-rich foods and avoid shopping when you're hungry to prevent impulse purchases.

3. Batch Cooking: Prepare larger portions of healthy meals and freeze them for future consumption. This reduces the need to order takeout or indulge in less healthy options when you're short on time.
4. Mindful Eating Space: Dedicate a specific space for mindful eating. Ensure it's free from distractions, comfortable, and conducive to savoring your meals.
5. Pre-Portion Snacks: If you enjoy having snacks available, portion them into individual servings. This prevents mindless overeating.
6. Mindful Snacking: Keep a variety of nutrient-rich snacks on hand for times when you need a quick bite. This reduces the likelihood of resorting to less nutritious options.
7. Stay Hydrated: Keep a water bottle within reach to stay hydrated throughout the day. Dehydration can sometimes trigger cravings.
8. Emotional Coping Tools: Have healthy coping mechanisms readily available, such as a journal for jotting down thoughts or a relaxation playlist for times of stress.
9. Create a Vision Board: Craft a vision board that includes images of your health and wellness goals. Place it in a visible area as a reminder of your aspirations.
10. Set Up Supportive Reminders: Use sticky notes, phone alarms, or digital reminders to prompt mindful eating practices and encourage healthier choices.
11. Engage Your Senses: Enhance your environment by engaging your senses. Use scented candles, calming music, or vibrant artwork to create a soothing atmosphere.
12. Limit Screen Time: Reduce exposure to food-related advertisements and images that can trigger cravings. Consider adjusting your social media feed to include more health-oriented content.

Overcoming Challenges in Creating a Supportive Environment

While modifying your environment can be empowering, it's important to anticipate and address challenges that may arise:

1. Resistance: Initially, you may encounter resistance to changing your environment. Start with small, manageable changes and gradually build upon them.
2. Social Pressure: When social situations encourage indulgence, communicate your health goals to friends and family. Seek out like-minded individuals who support your journey.
3. Relapse: There may be times when you give in to cravings despite your efforts. Remember that setbacks are normal. Reframe setbacks as learning opportunities and use them to refine your environment.

4. Lack of Time: Creating a supportive environment might feel overwhelming if you have a busy schedule. Start with one or two changes that align with your priorities.

Creating a supportive environment for success in craving control is a holistic approach that considers the physical and psychological factors that influence our choices. By thoughtfully modifying your surroundings, you can build a foundation that facilitates mindful and health-conscious eating. Whether it's stocking your kitchen with nutrient-rich foods, crafting a mindful eating space, or engaging social support, each step contributes to a more nurturing environment that empowers you to make mindful and intentional choices in the face of cravings. As you implement these strategies, remember that consistency is key, and every positive change you make brings you closer to your health and wellness goals.

Chapter Six

Mind-Body Approaches to Craving Control

•*Harnessing Meditation and Breathing Exercises*

In the quest for mindful and health-conscious eating, the power of the mind cannot be underestimated. Meditation and breathing exercises are valuable tools that can play a significant role in managing cravings and making intentional food choices. These practices tap into the mind-body connection, helping us become more attuned to our physical sensations, emotions, and thoughts. By incorporating meditation and breathing exercises into our routine, we can develop greater self-awareness, emotional regulation, and the ability to respond to cravings in a balanced and empowered manner. In this chapter, we delve into the benefits of meditation and breathing exercises for craving control and provide practical techniques for integrating these practices into your daily life.

Cravings often involve a complex interplay between physiological, psychological, and emotional factors. The mind plays a central role in how we perceive and respond to these factors. When we experience cravings, it's not just about the physical desire for a certain food; our thoughts and emotions are also involved. Meditation and breathing exercises offer a way to harness the power of the mind to navigate cravings with greater mindfulness and control.

Benefits of Meditation for Craving Control

1. Increased Awareness: Meditation cultivates awareness of your thoughts, feelings, and bodily sensations. This heightened awareness helps you recognize cravings as they arise, allowing you to respond mindfully rather than react impulsively.
2. Emotion Regulation: Cravings can be linked to emotional triggers. Meditation enhances your ability to observe and manage emotions without succumbing to them, reducing the likelihood of turning to food for emotional comfort.
3. Mindful Eating: Meditation supports mindful eating by encouraging you to savor each bite, fully experience the flavors, and tune in to your body's hunger and fullness cues.
4. Reduced Stress: Chronic stress can contribute to cravings. Meditation is a powerful stress-reduction tool that helps you manage stressors more effectively, reducing the likelihood of stress-driven cravings.
5. Delayed Gratification: Meditation enhances your ability to delay gratification, giving you the mental space to evaluate whether giving in to a craving aligns with your health goals.

Benefits of Breathing Exercises for Craving Control

1. Stress Reduction: Deep breathing exercises activate the body's relaxation response, reducing stress and anxiety. When stress is minimized, the likelihood of stress-induced cravings decreases.
2. Increased Oxygenation: Deep breathing increases oxygen levels in the body, promoting better circulation and oxygenation of tissues. This can positively impact brain function and decision-making.

3. Mind-Body Connection: Breathing exercises help you become more aware of the mind-body connection. You can notice how certain emotions and thoughts manifest as physical sensations, providing insights into triggers for cravings.
4. Focused Attention: Breathing exercises require focused attention on the breath. This practice enhances your ability to redirect your focus away from cravings and onto the present moment.

Practical Techniques for Integrating Meditation and Breathing Exercises

1. Mindful Breathing:
- Find a Comfortable Position: Sit or lie down in a comfortable position. Close your eyes and bring your attention to your breath.
- Focus on the Breath: Direct your attention to the sensation of your breath as it enters and leaves your body. Notice the rise and fall of your chest or the expansion and contraction of your abdomen.
- Counting Breaths: As you inhale, silently count "one." Exhale and count "two." Continue this pattern until you reach ten breaths, then start again from one. If your mind wanders, gently bring your focus back to the breath.

2. Body Scan Meditation:
- Begin with Breath Awareness: Start with a few minutes of mindful breathing to center yourself.
- Progressive Scan: Gradually bring your attention to different parts of your body, starting from your toes and moving up to your head. Notice any sensations without judgment.
- Observe Cravings: As you scan your body, observe if there are any sensations associated with cravings. Acknowledge these sensations and continue observing without reacting.

3. Loving-Kindness Meditation:

- Start with Breath Awareness: Begin by focusing on your breath to center yourself.
- Cultivate Loving-Kindness: Generate feelings of compassion and love for yourself. Silently repeat phrases like "May I be happy. May I be healthy. May I be at ease."
- Expand to Others: Gradually extend these wishes of well-being to loved ones, acquaintances, and even those with whom you have conflicts.

4.Box Breathing:

- Inhale: Inhale deeply through your nose for a count of four.
- Hold: Hold your breath for a count of four.

- Exhale: Exhale slowly and completely through your mouth for a count of four.
- Hold: Hold your breath for a count of four before inhaling again.
- Repeat: Continue this pattern for several breath cycles.

5. Diaphragmatic Breathing:
- Find a Comfortable Position: Sit or lie down with your back straight. Place one hand on your chest and the other on your abdomen.
- Inhale: Inhale deeply through your nose, allowing your abdomen to rise as you fill your lungs with air.
- Exhale: Exhale slowly through your mouth, feeling your abdomen fall.
- Focus on Your Breath: Keep your attention on the sensation of your breath moving in and out.

6. Breath Awareness during Cravings:
- Pause and Breathe: When a craving strikes, pause before taking any action. Take a few deep breaths to center yourself.
- Observe Sensations: As you breathe, notice any physical sensations associated with the craving. Observe without judgment.
- Label Emotions: Label any emotions that arise. For example, "I'm feeling anxious" or "I'm experiencing stress."
- Sustain the Breath: Continue deep breathing until the intensity of the craving subsides. This practice gives you the time and space to make a conscious choice about whether to indulge or choose a healthier option.

Integrating Meditation and Breathing into Your Routine

1. Morning Routine: Start your day with a few minutes of meditation or deep breathing. Set an intention for mindful eating and craving control.
2. Pre-Meal Practice: Before each meal, take a few moments to practice mindful breathing. This calms your mind and enhances your awareness of hunger and fullness cues.
3. Craving Moments: When a craving strikes, engage in a brief breathing exercise before deciding how to respond. This practice prevents impulsive decisions.
4. Evening Reflection: Dedicate a few minutes to meditation or deep breathing before bed. Reflect on your eating choices during the day and set intentions for the next day.
5. Mindful Eating Sessions: Combine meditation or breathing exercises with meals. Take a few mindful breaths before starting to eat and engage all your senses as you savor each bite.

Overcoming Challenges in Meditation and Breathing Practice

1. Inconsistency: Consistency is key to reaping the benefits of meditation and breathing exercises. Start with short sessions and gradually increase the duration as you build a routine.

2. Restless Mind: It's natural for your mind to wander during meditation. When you notice your mind wandering, gently bring your focus back to your breath or the meditation technique.
3. Time Constraints: If you're short on time, integrate short meditation or breathing exercises into your day, even if it's just for a few minutes.
4. Impatience: It takes time to experience the full benefits of these practices. Practice patience and approach the journey with an open mind.

Meditation and breathing exercises provide powerful tools for managing cravings and making intentional food choices. By cultivating awareness, regulating emotions, and fostering a mind-body connection, these practices empower you to respond to cravings with greater mindfulness and control. As you incorporate meditation and breathing exercises into your routine, remember that consistency and patience are key. Over time, you'll find that these practices become valuable resources for navigating the challenges of cravings and achieving a more balanced and health-conscious approach to eating.

•*Yoga and Physical Activity for Mental and Emotional Balance*

The intricate connection between the mind and body is undeniable. The choices we make in terms of physical activity can significantly impact our mental and emotional well-being. Engaging in activities such as yoga and regular exercise goes beyond the pursuit of physical fitness; it becomes a profound journey toward achieving mental clarity, emotional balance, and overall well-being. In this chapter, we delve into the benefits of yoga and physical activity for mental and emotional health, exploring how these practices promote stress reduction, mood enhancement, and a more harmonious relationship between the mind and body. We'll also provide practical guidance on incorporating these practices into your daily routine to harness their transformative potential.

The mind-body connection is a dynamic relationship that illustrates the influence of our mental and emotional states on our physical health, and vice versa. This connection means that our thoughts, emotions, and behaviors can influence the state of our physical body, while physical activities can impact our mental and emotional well-being. Engaging in activities that enhance this connection can lead to holistic wellness that encompasses the body, mind, and spirit.

The Power of Yoga for Mental and Emotional Health

Yoga is an ancient practice that combines physical postures, breath control, meditation, and ethical principles to promote well-being on multiple levels. The practice of yoga has gained popularity in modern times due to its remarkable ability to cultivate mental clarity, emotional resilience, and a sense of inner peace.

1. Stress Reduction: Yoga offers a sanctuary from the demands of daily life by creating a space for relaxation and inner reflection. Through gentle movement, breath awareness, and meditation, yoga activates the body's relaxation response, reducing the levels of stress hormones and promoting a sense of calm.
2. Mind-Body Awareness: Yoga encourages you to become attuned to the present moment, focusing on the sensations in your body and your breath. This heightened awareness enhances your ability to observe your thoughts and emotions without judgment, leading to a more balanced and mindful perspective.
3. Emotional Regulation: The practice of yoga involves exploring and releasing physical tension in the body, which can be linked to emotional tension. By targeting areas of physical discomfort, you can release stored emotions and develop tools for emotional regulation.
4. Mood Enhancement: Yoga stimulates the release of "feel-good" neurotransmitters such as endorphins and serotonin. This natural mood enhancement contributes to a more positive outlook and a greater sense of well-being.

Practical Techniques for Yoga Practice:

1. Beginner's Mind: Approach yoga with a beginner's mindset, letting go of expectations and judgments. Focus on the experience rather than achieving perfect poses.
2. Breath Awareness: Incorporate mindful breathing into your practice. Focus on deep, steady breaths that synchronize with your movements.
3. Gentle Movement: Begin with gentle, basic poses that allow you to explore your body's range of motion and gradually build strength and flexibility.
4. Mindful Meditation: Dedicate a few minutes to meditation at the beginning or end of your practice. Focus on your breath or a mantra to still the mind.
5. Progressive Relaxation: End your practice with a progressive relaxation exercise. Focus on releasing tension from each part of the body, promoting relaxation and inner calm.

Regular Exercise for Mental and Emotional Well-Being

Engaging in regular physical activity offers a multitude of benefits for mental and emotional health. Whether it's brisk walking, jogging, swimming, or dancing, any form of movement can contribute to stress reduction, improved mood, and enhanced cognitive function.

1. Stress Reduction: Exercise prompts the release of endorphins, which are natural stress reducers. Regular physical activity helps lower cortisol levels, reducing the body's stress response and promoting relaxation.
2. Mood Enhancement: Exercise has a direct impact on neurotransmitters that influence mood, such as dopamine and serotonin. These chemicals contribute to feelings of happiness, pleasure, and overall well-being.
3. Enhanced Cognitive Function: Physical activity increases blood flow to the brain, supporting cognitive function and mental clarity. It enhances focus, memory, and the ability to manage complex tasks.
4. Self-Confidence and Body Image: Engaging in regular exercise can improve self-esteem and body image. Achieving fitness goals and experiencing improvements in physical health can boost confidence and create a positive self-perception.

Practical Tips for Incorporating Physical Activity:

1. Choose Activities You Enjoy: Find physical activities that you genuinely enjoy, whether it's dancing, cycling, swimming, or hiking. When you enjoy the activity, you're more likely to stick with it.
2. Set Realistic Goals: Start with achievable goals and gradually increase the intensity and duration of your activities. This prevents burnout and supports consistency.
3. Create a Routine: Incorporate physical activity into your daily routine. This could be a morning walk, a lunchtime workout, or an evening yoga session.
4. Mix It Up: Variety prevents boredom and keeps you engaged. Combine different activities to challenge your body and mind in various ways.
5. Practice Mindful Movement: Approach physical activity with mindfulness. Focus on your breath, sensations, and the present moment as you move.

Overcoming Challenges in Yoga and Physical Activity

1. Time Constraints: If time is limited, break up your physical activity into shorter sessions throughout the day. Every bit of movement counts.
2. Lack of Motivation: Set small, achievable goals to overcome the initial lack of motivation. Once you experience the benefits, motivation often increases.
3. Physical Limitations: Choose activities that suit your fitness level and any physical limitations you may have. Consult a healthcare professional if needed.
4. Comparison: Avoid comparing yourself to others. Focus on your progress and celebrate your achievements, no matter how small.

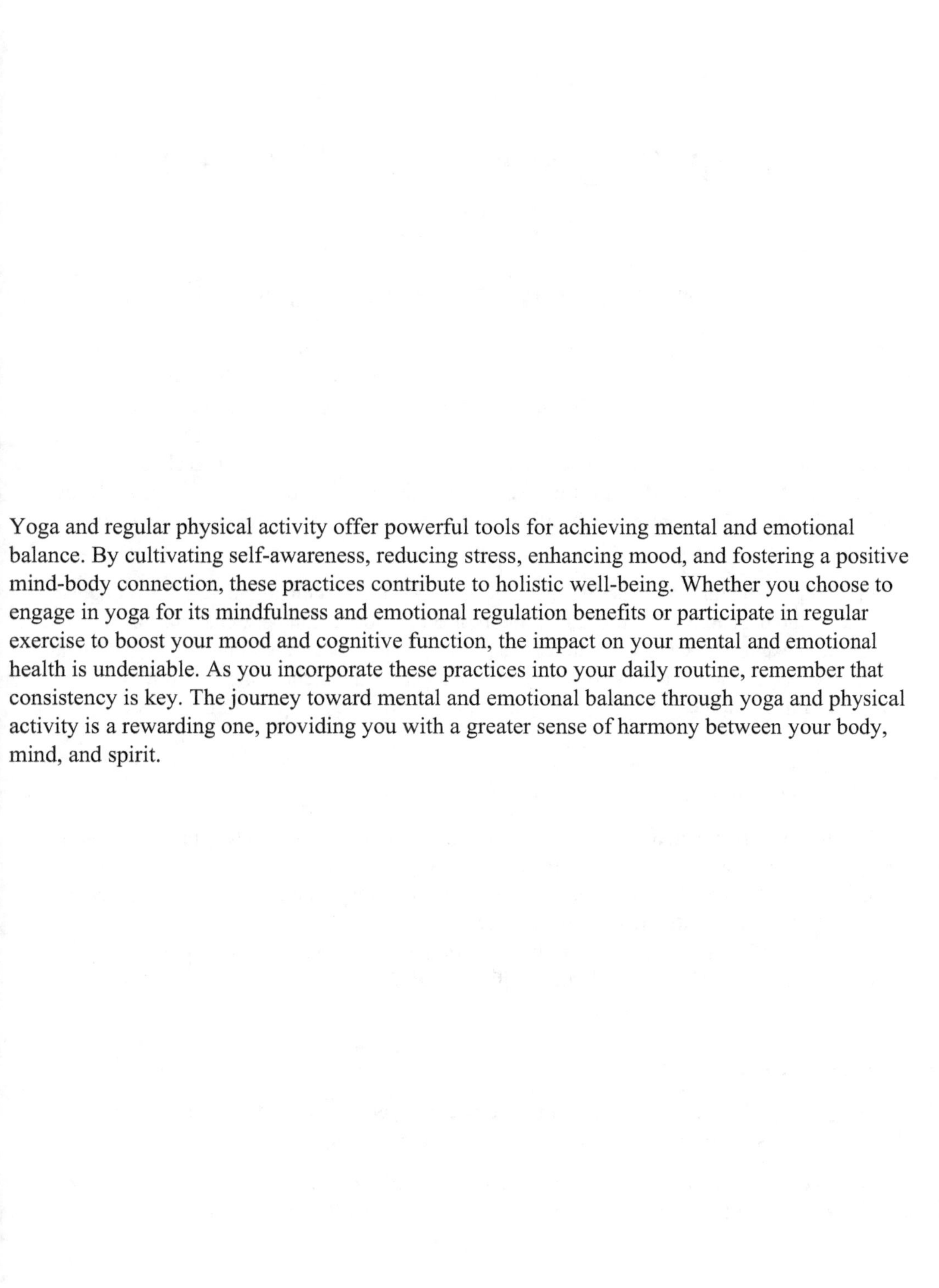

Yoga and regular physical activity offer powerful tools for achieving mental and emotional balance. By cultivating self-awareness, reducing stress, enhancing mood, and fostering a positive mind-body connection, these practices contribute to holistic well-being. Whether you choose to engage in yoga for its mindfulness and emotional regulation benefits or participate in regular exercise to boost your mood and cognitive function, the impact on your mental and emotional health is undeniable. As you incorporate these practices into your daily routine, remember that consistency is key. The journey toward mental and emotional balance through yoga and physical activity is a rewarding one, providing you with a greater sense of harmony between your body, mind, and spirit.

Chapter Seven
Navigating Social and Emotional Challenges

•*Dealing with Peer Pressure and Social Dining*

Navigating the realm of cravings and mindful eating becomes particularly intricate when peer pressure and social dining enter the picture. Social interactions often involve food, and the influence of friends, family, and colleagues can impact our food choices and eating behaviors. Dealing with peer pressure while striving to maintain control over cravings requires a delicate balance of assertiveness, self-awareness, and effective communication. In this chapter, we explore the challenges posed by peer pressure and social dining, offer strategies for asserting your health-conscious choices, and provide practical guidance on how to stay aligned with your cravings control goals even in social settings.

Peer pressure is the influence that friends, family, or peers exert on an individual's thoughts, behaviors, and decisions. While it's a common phenomenon, it can pose challenges when you're striving to make health-conscious choices, especially in the context of cravings and eating habits. Peer pressure can manifest in various ways, such as encouragement to indulge, criticism for making healthier choices, or feeling obliged to conform to the group's eating habits.

Social Influence and Food Choices:

1. Indulgence: Friends may encourage you to indulge in unhealthy foods, citing celebrations or special occasions as reasons to disregard your health goals.
2. Criticism: Making health-conscious choices can sometimes attract criticism or teasing from others who don't share the same perspective.
3. Conformity: The desire to fit in or avoid standing out can lead to conforming to the group's eating habits, even if they don't align with your goals.

Strategies for Dealing with Peer Pressure:

1. Stay Committed to Your Goals: Remind yourself of your health and well-being goals. Prioritize what's important to you over short-term peer influence.

2. Assertive Communication: Express your choices confidently without being confrontational. Use "I" statements to explain your decisions and avoid sounding judgmental.

3. Set Boundaries: Politely decline invitations or food offerings that don't align with your goals. Politely but firmly state that you're making mindful choices for your health.

4. Educate and Share: Educate your peers about your health goals and the importance of mindful eating. Share information that demonstrates your commitment to well-being.

5. Redirect Attention: Shift the focus from food to other aspects of the social interaction. Suggest engaging in an activity, conversation, or game.

6. Find Supportive Allies: Identify individuals who support your health goals and make an effort to spend time with them during social events.

Strategies for Maintaining Mindful Eating in Social Dining:

1. Preparation is Key: Before the event, review the menu or inquire about the food that will be served. Plan ahead and decide on healthier options.

2. Eat Mindfully: Pay attention to the taste, texture, and sensations of the food. Savor each bite and listen to your body's hunger and fullness cues.

3. Portion Control: Serve yourself smaller portions and avoid overloading your plate. You can always go for seconds if you're still hungry.

4. Prioritize Nutrient-Rich Foods: Choose foods that align with your health goals, such as lean proteins, vegetables, and whole grains.

5. Practice Moderation: Enjoy your favorite treats in moderation. Savor small portions and focus on the experience rather than quantity.

6. Stay Hydrated: Drink water throughout the meal to stay hydrated and support mindful eating.

Strategies for Navigating Social Pressures:

1. Anticipate Peer Influence: Be aware that social dining situations can trigger peer pressure. Mentally prepare to handle potential challenges.

2. Communicate Your Intentions: Inform your companions of your health-conscious choices. This prepares them and reduces potential pressure to indulge.

3. Lead by Example: Model mindful eating behaviors for others. Your positive actions might inspire them to make healthier choices too.

4. Be Firm but Polite: Politely decline offerings that don't align with your goals. Firmly but respectfully stand by your choices.

5. Shift the Focus: Initiate conversations that steer the focus away from food. Engage in discussions about shared interests or experiences.

6. Focus on Social Connection: Emphasize the importance of spending quality time with loved ones. Highlight the social aspect of the gathering rather than solely focusing on food.

Overcoming Challenges in Social Dining and Peer Pressure:

1. Fear of Standing Out: Remember that your health goals are valid and important. Don't let the fear of standing out deter you from making mindful choices.

2. Guilt and Obligation: Practice self-compassion and recognize that it's okay to prioritize your health. Release feelings of guilt and obligation.

3. Resisting Temptations: Visualize success and remind yourself of the rewards of staying aligned with your goals.

4. Handling Criticism: Embrace your choices with confidence. Understand that criticism may stem from others' insecurities.

Peer pressure and social dining can pose challenges to your cravings control journey, but with the right strategies and mindset, you can navigate these situations with confidence and success. Remember that your health and well-being are of utmost importance, and making mindful choices aligns with your long-term goals. Practicing assertive communication, setting boundaries, and prioritizing self-awareness can empower you to handle peer pressure effectively. In social dining scenarios, preparation, mindfulness, and moderation are your allies. By asserting your choices, focusing on your health, and leading by example, you can gracefully navigate social settings while staying committed to your health-conscious goals. The balance between social interactions and mindful eating is achievable, and with practice, it becomes a harmonious aspect of your cravings control journey.

•Coping with Stress and Emotional Triggers in Cravings Control

Stress and emotions are powerful influencers on our eating habits and cravings. From a demanding workday to relationship challenges, stressors and emotions can lead us to seek comfort in food, often resulting in impulsive and unhealthy choices. Learning how to cope with stress and manage emotional triggers is a crucial aspect of successful cravings control. In this

chapter, we explore the intricate connection between stress, emotions, and cravings, and provide practical strategies for effectively managing these triggers to make mindful and health-conscious choices.

The stress-eating connection is rooted in the intricate relationship between our emotions, hormones, and brain chemistry. When we experience stress, our bodies release hormones like cortisol, which can increase appetite and trigger cravings for high-calorie comfort foods. This biological response stems from our evolutionary survival mechanism, as stress was historically linked to the need for extra energy to handle life-threatening situations.

Impact of Emotional Triggers on Cravings:

1. Negative Emotions: Emotions such as anxiety, sadness, frustration, and loneliness can trigger cravings for foods that provide temporary comfort and pleasure.
2. Reward Center Activation: Comfort foods often trigger the brain's reward center, releasing feel-good neurotransmitters like dopamine, providing temporary relief from negative emotions.
3. Coping Mechanism: Consuming indulgent foods can serve as a coping mechanism to distract from or numb negative emotions temporarily.

Practical Strategies for Coping with Stress and Emotional Triggers:

Stress and emotional triggers can often lead to cravings for certain foods or substances as a way to cope with or escape from these feelings. However, it's important to find healthier ways to manage stress and emotional triggers to maintain overall well-being. Here are some practical strategies to help you cope with stress and emotional triggers of craving:

1. Identify your triggers: Take some time to reflect on the situations, emotions, or thoughts that tend to trigger your cravings. It could be stress, boredom, loneliness, or specific events. By understanding your triggers, you can develop strategies to address them.
2. Practice stress management techniques: Find healthy ways to manage stress, such as deep breathing exercises, meditation, yoga, or engaging in physical activity. These techniques can help reduce stress levels and alleviate the need for unhealthy coping mechanisms like food or substances.
3. Build a support system: Surround yourself with supportive friends, family, or a support group who can provide encouragement and understanding during challenging times. Sharing your feelings and experiences with others can help alleviate stress and prevent emotional triggers.

4. Engage in regular physical activity: Exercise is a great way to reduce stress, boost mood, and distract yourself from cravings. Find activities that you enjoy, whether it's going for a walk, dancing, cycling, or playing a sport. Regular physical activity can also improve your overall well-being and help you maintain a healthy lifestyle.
5. Practice mindful eating: When you feel the urge to indulge in cravings, pause and ask yourself if you're truly hungry or if it's an emotional craving. Practice mindful eating by

   paying attention to the taste, texture, and smell of your food. This can help you differentiate between physical hunger and emotional triggers.
6. Find alternative coping mechanisms: Discover healthy and enjoyable activities that can distract you from cravings. Engage in hobbies, listen to music, read a book, take a relaxing bath, or spend time in nature. Finding alternative coping mechanisms can help you redirect your focus and manage stress more effectively.
7. Plan and prepare healthy meals and snacks: By planning and preparing nutritious meals and snacks in advance, you can avoid impulsive and unhealthy food choices when cravings strike. Keep your kitchen stocked with wholesome options that satisfy your nutritional needs and help you maintain a balanced diet.
8. Get enough sleep: Lack of sleep can increase stress levels and make it more challenging to manage cravings. Aim for 7-9 hours of quality sleep each night to support your overall well-being

Managing Emotional Triggers and Cravings:

1. Pause and Reflect: When you feel the urge to indulge due to emotional triggers, pause for a moment. Take a few deep breaths and reflect on your feelings.
2. Mindful Awareness: Tune into your body and emotions. Ask yourself if you're truly hungry or if you're seeking comfort in food to cope with emotions.
3. Identify Triggers: Identify specific situations, people, or events that trigger emotional eating. Awareness allows you to create a plan to manage these triggers.
4. Find Healthy Alternatives: Replace food-based coping mechanisms with healthier alternatives. Engage in activities that bring you joy and provide emotional relief.
5. Practice Delayed Gratification: When a craving strikes, delay acting on it for a set amount of time. This pause gives you the opportunity to evaluate if you truly want the indulgence.
7. Mindful Consumption: If you choose to indulge, do so mindfully. Eat slowly, savor each bite, and pay attention to your body's signals of satisfaction.
8. Journal Your Triggers: Keep a journal where you record emotional triggers and the corresponding food cravings. This helps you recognize patterns and develop strategies.

Overcoming Challenges in Coping with Stress and Emotional Triggers:

1. Immediate Gratification: Recognize that indulging in comfort foods offers temporary relief but doesn't address the underlying emotions.

2. Fear of Emotions: Understand that emotions are natural and can be managed. Confronting them is a step toward growth and emotional well-being.
3. Impatience: Managing emotional triggers and cravings is a gradual process. Be patient with yourself as you learn new coping strategies.
4. Lack of Awareness: Cultivate self-awareness by regularly checking in with your emotions and identifying triggers. This practice enhances your ability to respond mindfully.

Coping with stress and emotional triggers is a vital aspect of successful cravings control. By developing strategies to manage stress and regulate emotions, you empower yourself to make mindful and health-conscious choices even in challenging situations. Engaging in stress management techniques, practicing emotion regulation, and adopting healthy alternatives to food-based coping mechanisms contribute to your overall well-being. As you incorporate these strategies into your daily routine, remember that it's a journey of self-discovery and growth. With time and practice, you'll find that you have the tools to navigate stress and emotions without turning to food for comfort. This shift in behavior not only supports your cravings control goals but also contributes to a more balanced and emotionally resilient life.

Chapter Eight

Customizing Your Craving Control Plan

•Developing Personalized Eating and Exercise Routines

Creating personalized eating and exercise routines is an essential step towards achieving long-term cravings control, weight management, and overall well-being. These routines empower you to make intentional and health-conscious choices that align with your unique preferences, lifestyle, and goals. In this chapter, we explore the importance of customization, offer guidance on crafting tailored eating and exercise routines, and provide practical tips for maintaining consistency and sustainability in your journey towards optimal health.

No one-size-fits-all approach to eating and exercise can cater to the diverse needs and preferences of individuals. Personalization acknowledges that each person's body, metabolism, preferences, and lifestyle are unique. By crafting routines that reflect your individuality, you increase the likelihood of adherence and success. Personalization encourages mindful choices, minimizes feelings of deprivation, and fosters a positive relationship with both food and exercise.

Customizing Your Eating Routine:

Customizing your eating routine can be a powerful tool in controlling cravings and promoting a healthy relationship with food. By tailoring your eating habits to your individual needs and preferences, you can create a sustainable and enjoyable approach to nourishing your body.

One way to customize your eating routine is by identifying and understanding your personal triggers for cravings. This could be certain foods, emotions, or situations that tend to lead to cravings. By recognizing these triggers, you can develop strategies to avoid or manage them effectively. For example, if stress is a trigger for you, finding alternative ways to cope with stress, such as practicing mindfulness or engaging in physical activity, can help reduce cravings.

Another important aspect of customizing your eating routine is considering your unique dietary needs and preferences. Everyone's nutritional requirements are different, so it's crucial to listen to your body and make choices that align with your individual needs. This could involve consulting with a registered dietitian or nutritionist to develop a personalized meal plan that takes into account any specific dietary restrictions or health conditions you may have.

In addition to considering your nutritional needs, it's also important to honor your food preferences. Restrictive diets or rigid eating plans can often lead to feelings of deprivation, which may increase the likelihood of cravings. Instead, focus on incorporating a variety of foods that you enjoy and that nourish your body. This can help create a positive and sustainable approach to eating, reducing the chances of feeling deprived and giving in to cravings.

Customizing your eating routine also involves establishing a structured eating schedule that works for you. This could mean eating three balanced meals a day, or incorporating smaller, more frequent meals and snacks throughout the day. Experiment with different eating patterns and listen to your body's hunger and fullness cues to find what works best for you. Having a consistent eating schedule can help regulate your blood sugar levels and prevent extreme hunger, which can contribute to cravings.

Furthermore, customizing your eating routine involves being mindful of portion sizes. It's important to be aware of how much you're eating and to practice portion control. This can be done by using smaller plates and bowls, measuring out serving sizes, and paying attention to your body's hunger and fullness signals. By being mindful of portion sizes, you can maintain a balanced and satisfying eating routine, reducing the likelihood of overeating and subsequent cravings.

Lastly, customizing your eating routine involves being flexible and allowing for occasional indulgences. Completely depriving yourself of foods you enjoy can often backfire and lead to intense cravings. Instead, allow yourself to enjoy

Crafting Your Exercise Routine:

Crafting your exercise routine is an essential step in achieving your fitness goals and maintaining a healthy lifestyle. By customizing your workout plan to fit your needs and preferences, you can make exercise enjoyable and sustainable.

First, consider your fitness goals. Are you looking to lose weight, build muscle, improve cardiovascular health, or simply stay active? Identifying your goals will help you determine the types of exercises you should incorporate into your routine. For example, if your goal is to build muscle, you may want to focus on strength training exercises. If weight loss is your goal, a combination of cardio and strength training may be more beneficial.

Next, consider your current fitness level. It's important to start at a level that is appropriate for your abilities and gradually progress as your fitness improves. If you're new to exercise, it may be helpful to consult with a fitness professional who can assess your fitness level and provide guidance on where to start. This will help prevent injury and ensure that you're challenging yourself enough to see progress.

When crafting your exercise routine, it's important to include a variety of exercises to target different muscle groups and provide a well-rounded workout. This can include cardiovascular exercises such as running, biking, or swimming, as well as strength training exercises like

weightlifting or bodyweight exercises. Additionally, incorporating flexibility exercises such as yoga or stretching can improve mobility and prevent injury.

Consider your schedule and availability when planning your exercise routine. Find a time of day that works best for you and try to stick to a consistent schedule. This will help establish a habit and make it easier to incorporate exercise into your daily routine. If time is limited, consider shorter, more intense workouts like high-intensity interval training (HIIT) to maximize your time and still get an effective workout.

Listen to your body and give yourself rest days. Rest and recovery are just as important as exercise itself. Overtraining can lead to injury and burnout, so it's crucial to allow your body time to rest and repair. Aim for at least one or two rest days per week to give your muscles time to recover and prevent overuse injuries.

Make your exercise routine enjoyable by incorporating activities that you genuinely enjoy. If you don't enjoy running, try a dance class or join a sports team. Experiment with different types of exercises until you find what you love. This will make it easier to stay motivated and consistent with your workouts.

Adjust your exercise routine as needed. As your fitness level improves, you may need to increase the intensity or duration of your workouts to continue seeing progress.

Tips for Developing a Personalized Routine:

Developing a personalized routine in eating and exercise is key to achieving your health and wellness goals. By tailoring your habits to your unique needs and preferences, you can create a sustainable lifestyle that promotes overall well-being. Here are some tips to help you get started:

1. Set clear goals: Before embarking on any changes, define your goals. Do you want to lose weight, gain muscle, improve your energy levels, or simply maintain a healthy lifestyle? Having specific goals will help you stay focused and motivated throughout your journey.

2. Consult a healthcare professional: If you have any underlying health conditions or specific dietary needs, it's essential to consult a healthcare professional or registered dietitian. They can provide personalized guidance based on your individual needs and help you create a safe and effective routine.
3. Understand your body's needs: Every person is unique, and what works for one may not work for another. Pay attention to your body's signals and learn to differentiate between hunger, thirst, and emotional cravings. Focus on providing your body with the nutrients it needs rather than following strict diets or trends.
4. Plan your meals: Meal planning is a great way to ensure you're consuming a balanced diet and avoiding impulsive or unhealthy food choices. Take some time each week to plan your meals and snacks, considering your nutritional needs and personal preferences. This will also help you save time and money by reducing food waste and unnecessary trips to the grocery store.

5. Prioritize whole foods: Incorporate a variety of whole, unprocessed foods into your diet. These include fruits, vegetables, lean proteins, whole grains, and healthy fats. These foods are nutrient-dense and provide your body with essential vitamins, minerals, and fiber.
6. Listen to your hunger and fullness cues: Practice mindful eating by paying attention to your body's hunger and fullness cues. Eat when you're hungry and stop when you're comfortably satisfied. This helps prevent overeating and promotes a healthy relationship with food.
7. Stay hydrated: Proper hydration is crucial for overall health and well-being. Aim to drink an adequate amount of water throughout the day and limit your consumption of sugary beverages. If you struggle with drinking enough water, try infusing it with fruits or herbs for added flavor.
8. Find an exercise routine you enjoy: Engaging in physical activity is essential for maintaining a healthy lifestyle. Find activities that you genuinely enjoy, whether it's running, dancing, swimming, or playing a sport. This will make it easier to stick to your routine and stay motivated.

Maintaining Sustainability and Adherence:

1. Set a Schedule: Create a weekly plan for meals and workouts. Having a structured routine makes it easier to stay on track.
2. Batch Cooking: Prepare meals in advance to save time and ensure you have nutritious options readily available.
3. Stay Hydrated: Drink plenty of water throughout the day to support digestion, energy levels, and overall well-being.
4. Seek Variety: Include a variety of foods and exercises to prevent boredom and ensure you're getting a diverse range of nutrients.
5. Practice Self-Compassion: Be kind to yourself and avoid self-criticism if you deviate from your routine occasionally.

6. Track Progress: Keep a journal to record your meals, workouts, and how you feel. Tracking progress can motivate and provide insights.
7. Celebrate Achievements: Acknowledge and celebrate your successes, whether they're related to weight loss, improved fitness, or healthier eating habits.

Overcoming Challenges in Personalized Routines:

1. Plateaus: If you hit a plateau in weight loss or fitness progress, adjust your routine by changing exercise intensity or trying new recipes.
2. Lack of Motivation: Revisit your goals, remind yourself of your reasons for making changes, and consider trying new activities or foods.
3. Time Constraints: Adapt your routine to fit your schedule. Even short workouts and quick, nutritious meals can have a positive impact.

4. External Pressures: Stay committed to your routine despite external influences. Communicate your goals to others to garner support.

Developing personalized eating and exercise routines is a transformative journey that empowers you to take control of your health and well-being. By tailoring your routines to your individual goals, preferences, and lifestyle, you set yourself up for sustainable success. Remember that personalization isn't about following strict rules but rather about creating a framework that aligns with your unique needs. As you embrace this journey, stay patient and open-minded. Progress may not always be linear, but with each mindful choice, you move closer to your aspirations. The power to create lasting change lies within your hands, and by customizing your eating and exercise routines, you're crafting a path to a healthier, happier, and more fulfilled life.

•Setting Realistic Goals and Tracking Progress

In the realm of health and wellness, few challenges are as universal as managing cravings. Whether it's the allure of sugary treats, the siren call of fast food, or the desire for salty snacks, cravings can be a formidable obstacle on the path to maintaining a balanced and healthy lifestyle. Setting realistic goals and effectively tracking progress play pivotal roles in overcoming these cravings, fostering better dietary choices, and achieving sustainable well-being. This extensive essay delves into the intricacies of cravings control, elucidates the importance of setting achievable objectives, and underscores the value of monitoring and evaluating progress in the context of managing cravings.

Cravings are intense desires for specific foods or substances that often defy rational decision-making. While the exact causes of cravings can vary, they often stem from a combination of physiological, psychological, and environmental factors. Factors such as hormonal imbalances, stress, boredom, and even conditioned responses can contribute to the emergence of cravings. The impact of unchecked cravings on health and well-being is multifaceted:

1. Nutritional Imbalance: Cravings frequently lead to the consumption of calorie-dense, nutrient-poor foods. This can disrupt the balance of essential nutrients in the body, leading to deficiencies and impairing overall health.
2. Weight Management: Succumbing to frequent cravings can sabotage weight management efforts. High-calorie, indulgent foods contribute to weight gain and hinder progress towards weight loss goals.

3. Emotional Well-being: Uncontrolled cravings often trigger feelings of guilt and shame, negatively impacting emotional well-being. This cycle of craving, indulgence, and subsequent regret can take a toll on mental health.
4. Long-Term Health: Consistently yielding to cravings, especially those for unhealthy foods, can increase the risk of chronic health conditions such as obesity, diabetes, and cardiovascular diseases.

Setting Realistic Goals in Cravings Control:

Setting realistic goals in cravings control is essential for individuals seeking to overcome addictive behaviors and maintain a healthy lifestyle. By establishing achievable and measurable objectives, individuals can stay motivated, track their progress, and make sustainable changes in their lives. Setting realistic goals helps individuals avoid feelings of failure or frustration, and instead fosters a sense of accomplishment and empowerment.

One of the first steps in setting realistic goals is to assess one's current situation and cravings patterns. This self-reflection allows individuals to understand the severity and frequency of their cravings, as well as the underlying triggers and factors contributing to them. By gaining insight into their cravings, individuals can set goals that are tailored to their specific needs and circumstances.

When setting goals, it is important to ensure that they are specific and measurable. Vague goals such as "reduce cravings" or "eat healthier" can be difficult to track and measure progress. Instead, individuals should establish clear and concrete objectives, such as "reduce daily cravings by 50%" or "consume at least five servings of fruits and vegetables each day." These specific goals provide individuals with a clear target to work towards and enable them to assess their progress accurately.

In addition to being specific and measurable, goals should also be realistic and attainable. It is important to set goals that are within reach and aligned with one's capabilities and resources. Setting unrealistic goals can lead to feelings of frustration and discouragement, which may ultimately hinder progress. By setting achievable goals, individuals can maintain a positive mindset and stay motivated throughout their journey.

To ensure that goals are realistic, individuals should consider their personal circumstances, such as their schedule, commitments, and available resources. For example, someone with a busy work schedule may find it more realistic to aim for three workouts per week instead of five. Taking into account these factors helps individuals set goals that are practical and can be integrated into their daily lives.

Another crucial aspect of setting realistic goals is breaking them down into smaller, manageable steps. Instead of aiming for a complete elimination of cravings, individuals can start by reducing cravings gradually. This approach allows for incremental progress and builds confidence along the way. Breaking goals into smaller steps also helps individuals identify specific actions they can take to work towards their larger objectives.

Furthermore, it is important to set timeframes for achieving goals. Without a deadline, goals can easily be postponed or forgotten. By setting a timeline, individuals create a sense of urgency and accountability for themselves. However, it is important to ensure that the timeframe is realistic and allows for steady progress. Rushing to achieve goals within an unreason

The Value of Tracking and Evaluating Progress:

Tracking and evaluating progress in craving control is an invaluable tool for individuals seeking to overcome addictive behaviors and maintain a healthy lifestyle. By actively monitoring and assessing one's progress, individuals can gain insight into their cravings, identify patterns and triggers, and make informed decisions to effectively manage and control cravings. This process empowers individuals to take charge of their cravings and make positive changes in their lives.

One of the primary benefits of tracking and evaluating progress in craving control is the ability to gain self-awareness. By keeping a record of cravings, individuals can identify common triggers or situations that lead to cravings. This self-awareness allows individuals to better understand the underlying causes of their cravings, such as stress, emotions, or environmental cues. With this knowledge, individuals can develop strategies to avoid or manage these triggers, reducing the likelihood of succumbing to cravings.

Tracking progress also provides individuals with a visual representation of their journey towards craving control. By documenting each craving and the corresponding actions taken to manage it, individuals can see their progress over time. This visual feedback serves as a powerful motivator, as individuals can witness their efforts paying off and their cravings becoming less frequent or intense. This reinforcement encourages individuals to continue their efforts and stay committed to their goals.

Additionally, tracking progress allows individuals to experiment with different strategies and evaluate their effectiveness. By recording the techniques used to manage cravings, individuals can identify which methods work best for them. For example, someone may find that deep breathing exercises or engaging in a hobby helps distract them from cravings, while others may benefit from talking to a supportive friend or engaging in physical activity. This knowledge enables individuals to refine their coping mechanisms and develop a personalized toolkit for craving control.

Furthermore, tracking progress provides individuals with a sense of accountability. By regularly reviewing their records, individuals can hold themselves accountable for their actions and decisions. This accountability helps individuals stay focused on their goals and make conscious choices to avoid triggers and manage cravings. It also serves as a reminder of the progress made and the importance of maintaining a healthy lifestyle.

In addition to personal accountability, tracking and evaluating progress can also be beneficial when seeking support from others. Sharing progress with a trusted friend, support group, or healthcare professional can provide individuals with encouragement, guidance, and constructive feedback. These external perspectives can offer valuable insights and suggestions for managing cravings, further enhancing the individual's progress.

Finally, tracking and evaluating progress in craving control allows individuals to celebrate their achievements, no matter how small. Each time an individual successfully manages a craving or implements a healthy coping mechanism, it is an accomplishment worth acknowledging.

Cravings control is a dynamic and multifaceted pursuit that demands a comprehensive approach. The significance of setting realistic goals and consistently tracking progress cannot be underestimated. By recognizing the complex interplay of physiological, psychological, and environmental factors contributing to cravings, individuals can tailor their goals to their unique circumstances. Armed with achievable objectives and a commitment to regular progress assessment, one can navigate the labyrinth of cravings with confidence and efficacy.

Remember, the journey to cravings control is not a linear path. It's a process characterized by victories and setbacks, moments of triumph and moments of struggle. Yet, armed with the power of setting realistic goals, progress tracking, and a steadfast resolve to cultivate healthy habits, individuals can overcome cravings, make informed dietary choices, and achieve a balanced and sustainable approach to wellness. In this pursuit, patience, self-compassion, and a willingness to learn from every step of the journey are invaluable allies on the road to lasting well-being.

Chapter Nine

Unlocking Lasting Weight Loss

•*The Connection Between Craving Control and Sustainable Weight Management*

Weight management has become a global concern due to the rising prevalence of obesity and related health issues. Achieving sustainable weight loss is often challenging, as it requires addressing various factors, including eating behaviors, physical activity, and psychological aspects. One crucial aspect that influences weight management is craving control. This essay aims to explore the connection between craving control and sustainable weight management, highlighting the impact of cravings on weight gain, the underlying causes of cravings, and effective strategies to manage them for long-term success.

Cravings refer to intense desires for specific foods, often high in sugar, fat, or salt content. These cravings can significantly contribute to weight gain as individuals tend to consume excessive calories beyond their energy needs. Research suggests that cravings are associated with the reward centers in the brain, leading to overeating and poor food choices. Moreover, studies have shown that individuals who frequently experience cravings are more likely to struggle with weight management and have a higher body mass index (BMI).

To effectively manage cravings, it is essential to comprehend their underlying causes. Biological factors play a significant role, such as hormonal imbalances, neurotransmitter activity, and genetic predispositions. Psychological factors, including stress, emotional eating, and learned behaviors, also contribute to cravings. Additionally, environmental factors like food availability, advertising, and social influence can trigger cravings. Understanding these causes helps individuals develop personalized strategies to control cravings and prevent weight gain.

Various strategies can aid in craving control and sustainable weight management. Firstly, adopting a balanced diet rich in fiber, protein, and healthy fats can help promote satiety and reduce cravings. Regular meal planning and incorporating nutritious snacks can prevent excessive hunger, which often leads to impulsive food choices. Mindful eating techniques, such as paying attention to hunger and fullness cues, can also enhance awareness of cravings and prevent overeating.

Moreover, stress management techniques, including exercise, meditation, and relaxation exercises, can reduce emotional eating triggers. Engaging in regular physical activity not only helps burn calories but also improves mood and reduces stress. Seeking support from a healthcare professional, registered dietitian, or joining support groups can provide guidance and accountability during the weight management journey.

Furthermore, cognitive-behavioral therapy (CBT) has been found effective in addressing the psychological aspects of cravings. CBT helps individuals identify and challenge negative thoughts and beliefs surrounding food, enabling them to develop healthier coping mechanisms. Additionally, techniques like distraction, substitution, and portion control can aid in managing cravings effectively.

Craving control is not a one-time solution but a lifelong commitment for sustainable weight management. Fad diets or extreme restrictions are often unsuccessful in the long run, as they do not address the root causes of cravings. Developing healthy eating habits, regular physical activity routines, and effective coping strategies are vital for maintaining weight loss and preventing relapse.

By learning to control cravings, individuals can establish sustainable habits that support long-term weight management. Here are some key points to consider:

1. Understand the nature of cravings: Cravings are intense desires for specific foods, often high in sugar, fat, or salt. They can be triggered by various factors, including emotions, stress, boredom, or even environmental cues. Recognizing that cravings are a normal part of human behavior can help individuals approach them with a balanced mindset.

2. Identify triggers: Take note of what triggers your cravings. Is it a specific time of day, a certain place, or certain emotions? Understanding your triggers can help you develop strategies to manage them effectively. For example, if you tend to crave unhealthy snacks in the evening while watching TV, consider finding alternative activities or stocking your pantry with healthier options.

3. Practice mindful eating: Mindful eating involves paying attention to your body's hunger and fullness cues. By slowing down, savoring each bite, and listening to your body, you can become more attuned to your true hunger and avoid overeating. Mindful eating also allows you to fully enjoy and appreciate the flavors and textures of your food.

4. Opt for balanced meals: Include a variety of nutrient-dense foods in your meals to promote satiety and reduce cravings. Focus on incorporating lean proteins, whole grains, fruits, vegetables, and healthy fats into your diet. These foods provide essential nutrients, fiber, and protein, which can help keep you feeling fuller for longer.

5. Stay hydrated: Dehydration can often be mistaken for hunger, leading to unnecessary snacking or overeating. Make sure to drink an adequate amount of water throughout the day to stay properly hydrated. If you find plain water boring, infuse it with fruits or herbs for added flavor.

6. Get enough sleep: Lack of sleep can disrupt hormone regulation and increase cravings for high-calorie, sugary foods. Aim for 7-9 hours of quality sleep each night to support your overall well-being and help manage cravings.

7. Manage stress: Stress can trigger emotional eating and cravings for comfort foods. Find healthy ways to manage stress, such as practicing yoga, meditation, or engaging in hobbies that bring you joy. If you find yourself turning to food for comfort, seek alternative forms of stress relief, such as talking to a friend, going for a walk, or engaging in a creative activity.

8. Plan and prepare meals: Having a well-thought-out meal plan and prepping meals in advance can help you make healthier choices and avoid impulsive, unhealthy food choices. Set aside

   time each week to plan your meals, create a grocery list, and prepare nutritious meals and snacks.

9. Incorporate regular physical activity: Exercise not only contributes to weight management but also helps regulate appetite and reduce cravings. Find physical activities that you enjoy and make them a regular part of your routine. Aim for a combination of cardiovascular exercises, strength training, and flexibility exercises for overall health and well-being.

10. Seek support: Surround yourself with a supportive network of friends, family, or a community with similar goals. Having someone to share your journey with, seek advice from, or simply vent to can make a significant difference in your ability to manage cravings and achieve sustainable weight management.

11. Remember, sustainable weight management is a long-term commitment that requires patience, consistency, and self-compassion. By understanding the connection between

craving control and sustainable weight management, you can develop strategies to overcome cravings and establish healthy habits that support your overall well-being.

In conclusion, the connection between craving control and sustainable weight management is undeniable. Cravings can significantly impact weight gain and hinder long-term success in weight management efforts. Understanding the underlying causes of cravings and implementing effective strategies can help individuals control their cravings and achieve sustainable weight loss. By adopting a holistic approach that focuses on nutrition, physical activity, psychological well-being, and long-term sustainability, individuals can overcome cravings and maintain a healthy weight for life.

•*Celebrating Victories and Overcoming Setbacks*

Craving control is an essential aspect of maintaining a healthy lifestyle and achieving weight management goals. It involves the ability to manage and redirect urges for specific foods that may be high in calories, sugar, fat, and salt. The journey of craving control is a dynamic one, marked by victories and setbacks. Celebrating victories and effectively overcoming setbacks in craving control is crucial for long-term success and well-being.

Cravings are intense desires for certain foods, often driven by a combination of physiological, psychological, and environmental factors. They can arise due to emotional triggers, stress, boredom, or the sight and smell of appetizing foods. Physiologically, the brain's reward center plays a pivotal role. When we indulge in foods high in sugar, fat, or salt, the brain releases dopamine, creating a pleasurable sensation and reinforcing the desire to consume these foods.

Understanding the intricate interplay between these factors is key to managing cravings effectively.

Celebrating Victories:

1. Recognizing Small Wins:

Craving control is a continuous battle, and every small victory counts. It is crucial to recognize and appreciate even the smallest achievements. Whether it's resisting the urge to indulge in a sugary treat or opting for a healthier snack instead, celebrating these small wins helps build confidence and reinforces the notion that we are capable of overcoming cravings.

2. Setting Milestones:

Setting milestones along the journey of craving control provides a sense of direction and purpose. These milestones can be personal goals such as going a week without giving in to cravings or reaching a certain weight loss target. When we achieve these milestones, it is essential to celebrate them as significant victories. This celebration can take the form of treating ourselves to something special or engaging in an activity that brings us joy.

3. Non-Food Rewards:

Often, our default mode of celebration involves indulging in food or drinks. However, when it comes to craving control, it is essential to find alternative ways to reward ourselves. Non-food rewards are equally effective and can help break the association between celebrations and unhealthy eating habits. Examples of non-food rewards include treating yourself to a spa day, buying a new book or gadget, or taking a day off to relax and engage in activities you enjoy.

4. Social Support and Accountability:

Celebrating victories in craving control becomes even more meaningful when shared with others. Engaging in a support system, whether it's with friends, family, or a community, can provide a sense of accountability and encouragement. Sharing your achievements with others who understand the struggle can make the celebration more meaningful and help you stay motivated on your journey.

5. Documenting Progress:

Keeping track of your progress is an effective way to celebrate victories in craving control. Documenting your achievements, whether it's through a journal, a mobile app, or a visual representation, allows you to reflect on how far you've come. Seeing your progress visually can be incredibly motivating and serves as a reminder of the victories

Overcoming Setbacks:

1. Self-Reflection and Understanding:

When faced with a setback, it's crucial to take a step back and reflect on what led to the slip-up. Understanding the triggers, emotions, or situations that caused the setback can help us identify patterns and make necessary adjustments. By gaining insight into our cravings and the circumstances surrounding them, we can develop strategies to prevent similar setbacks in the future.

2. Cultivating Self-Compassion:

Setbacks can often lead to feelings of guilt, shame, or disappointment. It's important to practice self-compassion during these times and remember that we are human. Acknowledge that setbacks are a normal part of the process and that everyone experiences them. Treat yourself with kindness and understanding, just as you would a friend who is going through a similar situation.

3. Reframing Setbacks as Learning Opportunities:

Instead of viewing setbacks as failures, reframe them as valuable learning opportunities. Each setback can provide insights into our triggers, weaknesses, and areas that require further attention. Embrace setbacks as chances to grow, adapt, and refine your approach to craving control. Use the knowledge gained from setbacks to develop new strategies and strengthen your commitment to your goals.

4. Revisiting Goals and Creating Action Plans:

Setbacks may indicate that our initial goals or action plans need adjustment. Take the time to reassess your goals and make sure they are realistic, attainable, and aligned with your overall well-being. Break down your goals into smaller, manageable steps and create action plans that outline specific actions you can take to overcome cravings. Having a clear roadmap will help you regain focus and motivation.

5. Seeking Support:

During times of setbacks, seeking support from others can provide invaluable guidance and encouragement. Reach out to friends, family, or a support group who understand your journey and can offer empathy, advice, and motivation. Sharing your struggles and successes with others who can relate can help you feel less alone and more motivated to overcome setbacks.

6. Practicing Mindfulness and Stress Management (continued):

Setbacks in craving control can sometimes be triggered by stress, anxiety, or other negative emotions. Incorporating mindfulness and stress management techniques into your daily routine can help you navigate these challenges more effectively. Engage in activities such as meditation, deep breathing exercises, or yoga to cultivate a sense of calm and reduce stress levels. By managing stress proactively, you can minimize the likelihood of setbacks and maintain control over your cravings.

7. Celebrating Small Victories:

Even in the face of setbacks, it's important to acknowledge and celebrate the small victories along the way. Recognize and appreciate the progress you have made, no matter how small it may seem. By focusing on the positive aspects of your journey, you can maintain a sense of motivation and resilience, which will help you overcome setbacks more effectively.

8.   Staying Persistent and Patient:

Overcoming setbacks in craving control requires persistence and patience. Understand that progress is not always linear, and setbacks are a natural part of the process. Stay committed to your goals and remember that each setback is an opportunity to learn, grow, and become stronger. Trust in yourself and your ability to overcome challenges, and keep moving forward with determination.

Setbacks in craving control are inevitable, but they do not define your journey. By practicing self-reflection, self-compassion, and resilience, you can overcome setbacks and regain control over your cravings. Remember to seek support, revisit your goals, and celebrate small victories along the way. Stay persistent, patient, and committed to your well-being, and you will bounce back stronger than ever before.

Long-Term Strategies:

1.   Consistency: Consistency is key to both celebrating victories and overcoming setbacks. Keep practicing craving control strategies even after achieving your initial goals.
2.   Adaptability: The journey of craving control is not linear. Be adaptable and willing to modify your approach as you learn more about your triggers and responses.
3.   Lifestyle Changes: Focus on making sustainable lifestyle changes rather than temporary fixes. Gradual adjustments are more likely to lead to lasting results.
4.   Positive Environment: Surround yourself with a positive and supportive environment that aligns with your goals. This includes both physical spaces and the people you interact with.
5.   Professional Help: If craving control becomes overwhelming or interferes with your overall well-being, consider seeking guidance from a registered dietitian, therapist, or counselor.

The journey of craving control is marked by a series of victories and setbacks. It's essential to celebrate each victory, no matter how small, as they signify progress and growth. Equally important is the ability to overcome setbacks with resilience, self-compassion, and a determination to continue moving forward. The process of managing cravings is dynamic and requires ongoing effort, self-awareness, and a willingness to learn from both successes and challenges. By adopting a positive mindset, embracing a supportive environment, and seeking professional guidance when needed, individuals can navigate the complex terrain of craving control and achieve sustainable success in their health and well-being goals.

Chapter Ten
Embracing a New Energetic You

•*Reaping the Benefits of Improved Energy and Vitality*

Craving control is a central component of a healthy lifestyle, influencing our dietary choices, weight management efforts, and overall well-being. While the immediate goal of craving control is to resist the allure of unhealthy foods, the benefits extend far beyond just avoiding indulgence. One of the significant rewards of successful craving control is the substantial improvement in energy levels and overall vitality. By understanding how craving control affects energy and vitality, individuals can harness these benefits to enhance their quality of life and achieve their wellness goals.

The Relationship Between Cravings and Energy:

Cravings are powerful urges for specific foods that often carry high caloric content and low nutritional value. These foods, laden with sugars, fats, and salts, can provide quick bursts of energy but are typically followed by energy crashes. The consumption of high-sugar foods leads to rapid spikes in blood sugar levels, causing a subsequent crash that leaves individuals feeling fatigued, irritable, and craving more sugary treats. This cycle of energy spikes and crashes is detrimental to overall well-being and can hinder productivity and mood.

Vicious Cycle of Cravings and Energy:

The relationship between cravings and energy forms a vicious cycle. Cravings lead to the consumption of unhealthy foods, which result in energy spikes followed by crashes. These crashes trigger additional cravings, often for the same unhealthy foods, perpetuating the cycle. Over time, this pattern not only affects physical health but also takes a toll on mental and emotional well-being. Breaking this cycle through effective craving control can have a transformative impact on energy levels and vitality.

Benefits of Improved Energy and Vitality:

1. Sustained Energy: Successful craving control involves making conscious choices to consume balanced, nutrient-dense foods. These foods provide a steady and sustained release of energy throughout the day, preventing the energy roller coaster caused by indulging in sugary and processed snacks.

2. Enhanced Mood: Stable blood sugar levels resulting from healthier food choices contribute to stable moods. Balanced energy levels reduce irritability and mood swings often associated with sugar crashes, promoting emotional well-being.

3. Improved Cognitive Function: Proper nourishment supports brain health, enhancing cognitive functions such as focus, concentration, and memory. Steady energy levels prevent brain fog caused by rapid fluctuations in blood sugar.

4. Optimized Physical Performance: Nutrient-rich foods fuel physical activities by providing the necessary energy without the crashes associated with unhealthy choices. This allows for improved endurance, strength, and overall performance.

5. Better Sleep: Cravings for unhealthy foods, especially close to bedtime, can disrupt sleep patterns. Improved craving control minimizes nighttime overeating, leading to better sleep quality and overall restfulness.

6. Weight Management: Effective craving control contributes to weight management by reducing consumption of high-calorie, low-nutrient foods. Maintaining a healthy weight is linked to improved energy levels and reduced risk of chronic conditions.

Strategies for Reaping the Benefits:

1. Balanced Meals: Prioritize balanced meals that include a combination of complex carbohydrates, lean proteins, and healthy fats. This combination provides sustained energy and promotes satiety.

2. Frequent Meals: Opt for smaller, more frequent meals and snacks throughout the day. This approach prevents extreme hunger and the subsequent tendency to make impulsive, unhealthy choices.

3. Whole Foods: Choose whole, unprocessed foods over refined and packaged options. Whole foods provide essential nutrients, vitamins, and minerals that support overall health and vitality.

4. Hydration: Staying hydrated is crucial for maintaining energy levels. Dehydration can lead to feelings of fatigue and confusion, often mistaken for hunger or cravings.

5. Mindful Eating: Engage in mindful eating practices to connect with hunger and fullness cues. This helps prevent overeating and promotes conscious choices about food consumption.

6. Nutrient-Dense Snacks: Keep nutrient-dense snacks, such as fresh fruits, vegetables, nuts, and seeds, readily available to satisfy hunger between meals and prevent energy crashes.

7. Regular Physical Activity: Incorporate regular physical activity into your routine. Exercise boosts energy levels, enhances mood, and reduces the likelihood of turning to comfort foods for emotional reasons.

8. Sleep Routine: Prioritize sleep hygiene by maintaining a consistent sleep schedule and creating a conducive sleep environment. Quality sleep is essential for energy restoration.

9. Stress Management: Implement stress-reduction techniques such as meditation, deep breathing, and yoga to prevent stress-induced cravings and maintain balanced energy levels.

10. Accountability and Support: Share your craving control goals with friends, family, or a support group. Having a support system can provide encouragement and motivation to stay on track.

The journey of craving control extends far beyond resisting unhealthy foods. It encompasses a broader perspective on energy management and overall vitality. By reaping the benefits of improved energy levels, stable moods, and enhanced cognitive and physical performance, individuals can achieve a higher quality of

life. The connection between craving control and energy is profound, influencing both immediate well-being and long-term health outcomes. Embracing strategies that prioritize balanced nutrition, mindful eating, regular physical activity, and stress management empowers individuals to break free from the vicious cycle of cravings and energy crashes. As a result, they can experience sustained energy, heightened vitality, and a renewed sense of well-being that propels them toward their wellness goals.

•*Maintaining Your Craving Control Skills for the Long Term*

Achieving successful craving control is a significant accomplishment that requires dedication, self-awareness, and the development of effective strategies. However, the journey doesn't end once you've mastered these skills. Maintaining your craving control abilities for the long term is equally, if not more, important. Sustaining your progress ensures that the benefits you've gained in terms of health, well-being, and overall quality of life continue to flourish. In this exploration, we delve into the nuances of maintaining craving control skills for the long term and offer practical insights to support your ongoing success.

While achieving initial craving control goals can be challenging, maintaining those achievements over the long term presents its own set of obstacles. Life is full of changes, stressors, and temptations that can test even the most robust craving control skills. Additionally, complacency and a sense of achievement can lead to a relaxation of efforts, making it easier to revert to old habits. To counter these challenges, adopting a proactive and adaptable approach is essential.

Mindset for Long-Term Success:

1. Continuous Improvement: Embrace the philosophy of continuous improvement. Rather than resting on past achievements, view each day as an opportunity to refine your craving control skills and make incremental progress.
2. Growth Mindset: Cultivate a growth mindset that thrives on challenges and treats setbacks as learning experiences. This mindset fosters resilience and a willingness to adapt and improve over time.
3. Patience and Persistence: Understand that long-term success requires patience and persistence. Changes in habits take time to solidify, and setbacks are a natural part of the journey.
4. Self-Compassion: Be kind to yourself throughout the process. Acknowledge that slip-ups may occur, but don't let them define your progress. Treat yourself with the same compassion you would offer a friend.

Strategies for Long-Term Maintenance:

1. Regular Self-Assessment: Continuously evaluate your craving control skills and behaviors. Reflect on your progress, identify areas that need improvement, and celebrate your successes.
2. Setting New Goals: As you achieve your initial craving control goals, set new ones to keep yourself motivated and engaged. These goals can be related to specific foods, portion control, or broader wellness objectives.
3. Variety in Food Choices: While maintaining a balanced and nutritious diet, explore new foods and recipes to prevent boredom. Variety not only enhances the pleasure of eating but also prevents monotony that could lead to craving relapses.

4. Mindful Eating Practice: Continue practicing mindful eating to stay connected with hunger and satiety cues. Mindful eating helps prevent overeating and ensures you make conscious choices.
5. Regular Physical Activity: Maintain a consistent exercise routine. Physical activity not only supports craving control but also contributes to overall well-being, energy levels, and weight management.
6. Stress Management: Keep stress in check through relaxation techniques, hobbies, and activities that bring joy. Stress can trigger emotional eating, so managing it is essential for long-term success.
7. Sleep Prioritization: Ensure you prioritize sufficient, quality sleep. Sleep deprivation can disrupt hormones that regulate hunger and cravings, making it harder to maintain control.
8. Social Support: Surround yourself with individuals who support your healthy habits. Engaging in social activities that don't revolve around food can help maintain progress.
9. Tracking and Accountability: Continue using tools like food journals or tracking apps to monitor your eating patterns. Accountability can prevent complacency and offer insights into areas needing improvement.
10. Celebrate Non-Scale Wins: Focus on non-scale victories, such as improved mood, increased energy, and enhanced self-esteem. These wins reinforce the positive effects of your efforts beyond just weight-related goals.
11. Professional Guidance: Consider periodic check-ins with a registered dietitian, therapist, or counselor. These professionals can provide guidance, address challenges, and offer personalized strategies for long-term success.
12. Adaptability: Be open to adjusting your strategies as circumstances change. Life events, schedules, and preferences evolve, so your craving control approach should be adaptable as well.

Maintaining your craving control skills for the long term requires dedication, self-awareness, and an adaptable mindset. The journey is not a linear path; it's marked by both successes and setbacks. By cultivating a growth mindset, setting new goals, practicing mindfulness, and prioritizing overall well-being, you can navigate the challenges that arise and continue to reap the rewards of your efforts. Remember that the benefits extend beyond the surface—better energy, mood, and vitality are all part of the ongoing journey. Embrace the process, celebrate your victories, and commit to nurturing your craving control skills as an integral part of your holistic approach to health and wellness.

Chapter Eleven

Recipes for Craving-Busting Delights

•*Nourishing and Delicious Meals to Satisfy and Sustain*

The relationship between food cravings and the pursuit of a healthy lifestyle is often seen as conflicting. However, it's possible to strike a balance by creating meals that both satisfy your cravings and provide the nourishment your body needs. Nourishing and delicious meals can play a significant role in managing cravings, promoting satiety, and sustaining your overall well-being. By understanding the principles of crafting such meals, you can embark on a culinary journey that brings satisfaction without compromising your health goals.

Balancing Cravings and Nutrition:

The key to creating meals that satisfy both your cravings and nutritional requirements lies in finding harmony between flavors, textures, and nutrient content. This approach challenges the notion that healthy meals are bland and unsatisfying. Instead, it embraces the concept of nourishing your body with nutrient-rich ingredients while indulging your taste buds with flavors and textures that satisfy your cravings.

Components of Nourishing and Delicious Meals:

1. Complex Carbohydrates: Incorporate complex carbohydrates like whole grains (quinoa, brown rice, whole wheat pasta) that provide sustained energy, support blood sugar control, and keep you full longer.
2. Lean Proteins: Include lean protein sources such as chicken, turkey, fish, tofu, beans, and legumes. Protein promotes satiety, supports muscle health, and aids in managing cravings.
3. Healthy Fats: Incorporate sources of healthy fats like avocados, nuts, seeds, and olive oil. Healthy fats add richness to meals, enhance flavors, and provide a sense of satisfaction.

4. Vibrant Vegetables: Prioritize a variety of colorful vegetables in your meals. Vegetables provide essential vitamins, minerals, and fiber while adding texture and visual appeal.
5. Flavorful Herbs and Spices: Use a diverse range of herbs and spices to elevate flavors without relying heavily on salt and unhealthy condiments.
6. Natural Sweeteners: Choose natural sweeteners like honey, maple syrup, or fresh fruits to satisfy sweet cravings without the negative effects of refined sugars.

Strategies for Crafting Nourishing and Delicious Meals:

1. Balance and Moderation: Instead of completely avoiding foods you crave, incorporate them in moderation within a balanced meal. This prevents feelings of deprivation and minimizes the likelihood of overindulgence.
2. Meal Planning: Plan your meals ahead of time to ensure you have the necessary ingredients to create balanced dishes. This prevents last-minute decisions driven by cravings.
3. Mindful Eating: Practice mindful eating to fully savor and appreciate the flavors, textures, and aromas of your meals. This approach can enhance satisfaction and reduce the urge to overeat.
4. Experimentation: Embrace culinary experimentation by trying new ingredients, recipes, and cooking techniques. This keeps meals exciting and prevents monotony.
5. Preparation Techniques: Opt for cooking methods that retain the nutritional value and flavors of ingredients, such as roasting, steaming, grilling, or sautéing with minimal oil.

6. Portion Control: Pay attention to portion sizes to avoid excessive calorie consumption. Even nutrient-dense foods should be enjoyed in appropriate quantities.

Nourishing and Delicious Meal Ideas:

1. Quinoa and Vegetable Stir-Fry: A combination of quinoa, stir-fried vegetables, and lean protein (tofu, chicken, or shrimp) seasoned with soy sauce, ginger, and garlic creates a flavorful, nutrient-rich meal.

2. Mediterranean Bowl: Build a bowl with mixed greens, cherry tomatoes, cucumber, olives, feta cheese, grilled chicken or chickpeas, and a drizzle of olive oil and balsamic vinegar.

3. Whole Wheat Pasta Primavera: Whole wheat pasta tossed with sautéed bell peppers, zucchini, cherry tomatoes, and grilled chicken, all dressed in a light olive oil and herb sauce.

4. Sweet Potato and Black Bean Tacos: Load whole grain tortillas with roasted sweet potatoes, black beans, avocado slices, salsa, and a sprinkle of cheese for a satisfying taco feast.

5. Oatmeal Parfait: Layer Greek yogurt, mixed berries, and granola for a nutrient-packed breakfast or snack that balances sweetness with protein and fiber.

6. Veggie Omelette: Whisk eggs with a splash of milk, then fill the omelette with sautéed spinach, mushrooms, and feta cheese for a protein-rich, savory meal.

7. Homemade Pizza: Create a whole wheat pizza crust topped with tomato sauce, mozzarella cheese, and a variety of colorful vegetables. Add lean protein if desired.

8. Chia Seed Pudding: Mix chia seeds with almond milk, a touch of honey, and vanilla extract. Top with fresh fruit, nuts, and seeds for a nutritious and indulgent dessert.

Crafting nourishing and delicious meals that satisfy and sustain cravings is a creative endeavor that balances flavor, nutrition, and satisfaction. By incorporating complex carbohydrates, lean proteins, healthy fats, and an array of colorful vegetables, you can create dishes that cater to both your taste buds and your body's nutritional needs. Embrace a mindful approach to eating, experiment with different ingredients, and maintain a balance between indulgence and moderation. Ultimately, mastering the art of crafting nourishing and delicious meals empowers you to savor food while supporting your long-term health and wellness goals.

•*Smart Snack Ideas to Tame the Midday Munchies*

The midday munchies, that familiar feeling of hunger between meals, often lead to snack choices that may not align with your health and wellness goals. However, with thoughtful planning, you can turn snack time into an opportunity to nourish your body, control cravings, and sustain your energy levels throughout the day. Smart snack ideas encompass a combination of nutrient-rich ingredients that satisfy your hunger while providing essential vitamins, minerals, and energy. In this exploration, we'll delve into creative and practical snack options that effectively tame the midday munchies.

The Importance of Smart Snacking:

Smart snacking serves as a bridge between meals, helping to regulate blood sugar levels, preventing overeating during main meals, and providing essential nutrients for sustained energy. It's an opportunity to curb hunger and cravings while supporting overall well-being. The key is to choose snacks that strike a balance between satiety, flavor, and nutrition.

Elements of Smart Snack Choices:

1. Protein: Including a source of protein in your snacks promotes fullness and helps stabilize blood sugar levels. Protein-rich snacks can include nuts, seeds, Greek yogurt, cottage cheese, lean meats, and legumes.
2. Fiber: Fiber contributes to feelings of satiety and aids in digestion. Fiber-rich snacks can include fruits, vegetables, whole grains, and nuts.
3. Healthy Fats: Healthy fats provide a sense of satisfaction and contribute to the overall nutrient profile of your snack. Options include avocados, nuts, seeds, and olive oil.
4. Complex Carbohydrates: Complex carbohydrates provide sustained energy and prevent rapid blood sugar spikes. Whole grains, fruits, and vegetables are excellent sources.
5. Portion Control: Mindful portion control is crucial for snacking. Aim for balanced portions that satisfy your hunger without causing overconsumption of calories.

Smart Snack Ideas:

1. Apple Slices with Nut Butter: Pair apple slices with a dollop of almond or peanut butter. The combination of fiber from the apple and healthy fats from the nut butter creates a satisfying snack.
2. Greek Yogurt Parfait: Layer Greek yogurt with mixed berries and a sprinkle of granola or nuts for a protein-packed snack rich in antioxidants and probiotics.
3. Carrot Sticks and Hummus: Enjoy baby carrot sticks with a side of hummus. The crunchiness of the carrots and the creaminess of the hummus create a delightful contrast.
4. Trail Mix: Create a custom trail mix with a variety of nuts, seeds, and dried fruits. This snack provides a balance of healthy fats, protein, and natural sugars.
5. Hard-Boiled Egg with Whole Grain Crackers: Pair a hard-boiled egg with whole grain crackers for a protein and fiber-rich snack that satisfies hunger and provides essential nutrients.
6. Air-Popped Popcorn: Opt for air-popped popcorn seasoned with a sprinkle of nutritional yeast or your favorite herbs. It's a light and crunchy snack that's low in calories.
7. Cottage Cheese and Pineapple: Enjoy cottage cheese with a side of fresh pineapple chunks. This combination offers a mix of protein, vitamins, and natural sweetness.

8. Chia Seed Pudding: Make chia seed pudding using almond milk, chia seeds, and a touch of honey or maple syrup. Top with berries for added flavor and nutrients.
9. Whole Grain Toast with Avocado: Top whole grain toast with mashed avocado, a sprinkle of red pepper flakes, and a drizzle of olive oil. This snack provides healthy fats and fiber.
10. Homemade Veggie Chips: Create your own veggie chips by thinly slicing vegetables like sweet potatoes, zucchini, or kale, then baking them until crispy.
11. Frozen Grapes: Freeze grapes for a refreshing and naturally sweet snack that satisfies cravings for something cold and sweet.
12. Mini Wrap: Fill a small whole wheat tortilla with lean turkey, lettuce, tomato, and a smear of mustard for a balanced and satisfying mini wrap.
13. Berries and Cottage Cheese: Mix fresh berries with cottage cheese for a snack rich in antioxidants, protein, and vitamins.
14. Edamame: Enjoy a serving of steamed edamame sprinkled with sea salt for a protein-packed and satisfying snack.
15. Nutrient-Rich Smoothie: Blend together spinach, banana, almond milk, and a scoop of protein powder for a nutrient-rich and filling smoothie.

Smart snack ideas are an essential part of a balanced and healthy diet. By choosing snacks that combine protein, fiber, healthy fats, and complex carbohydrates, you can effectively tame the midday munchies while providing your body with essential nutrients and sustained energy. Snacking should never be seen as an excuse to indulge in unhealthy options; instead, it's an opportunity to nourish your body and support your overall well-being. With these creative and practical snack ideas, you can make informed choices that contribute to your health and wellness goals. Remember, the key is balance, variety, and mindfulness when it comes to snacking.

Chapter Twelve
Conclusion

•*Reflecting on Your Journey to Craving Control*

The journey to craving control is a transformative experience that involves self-discovery, self-discipline, and a commitment to better health. As you navigate the complexities of managing your cravings and making healthier food choices, taking time to reflect on your journey is a valuable practice. Reflection not only allows you to appreciate your progress but also offers insights into your challenges, victories, and the strategies that have worked best for you. In this exploration, we delve into the importance of reflection, the benefits it brings, and how to effectively integrate it into your ongoing quest for craving control.

The Value of Reflection:

Reflection is a conscious and deliberate process of examining your thoughts, actions, and experiences. It's an opportunity to look back on your journey to craving control, celebrate your achievements, and learn from your setbacks. Reflection offers the following benefits:

1. Self-Awareness: Reflecting helps you gain a deeper understanding of your triggers, behaviors, and emotions related to cravings. This self-awareness is essential for making informed choices.
2. Celebration of Progress: Acknowledging how far you've come in your craving control journey boosts your confidence and motivation to continue your efforts.
3. Learning from Setbacks: Reflection allows you to identify patterns that lead to setbacks. Learning from these experiences helps you develop strategies to overcome similar challenges in the future.
4. Adaptation: As you reflect on your journey, you can adapt your strategies based on what's working and what isn't. This flexibility enhances your chances of long-term success.
5. Motivation: Reflecting on your successes and the positive changes you've experienced serves as a powerful source of motivation to keep moving forward.

Ways to Reflect on Your Craving Control Journey:

1. Journaling: Keeping a craving control journal can be a therapeutic and insightful practice. Write about your daily experiences, challenges, victories, emotions, and the strategies you've used.
2. Mindful Eating: Practice mindful eating during meals and snacks. Reflect on the flavors, textures, and sensations you experience. This practice can foster a deeper connection to your body's signals.
3. Weekly Reviews: Set aside time each week to review your progress. Consider what went well, what could be improved, and how you managed your cravings. This practice helps you stay on track.
4. Visual Reminders: Create visual reminders of your progress, such as before-and-after photos, a food journal, or a vision board. These reminders can be powerful motivators.
5. Support Group Sharing: If you're part of a craving control support group, sharing your experiences with others can offer fresh perspectives and insights.

Reflective Questions for Your Journey:

1. What Triggers My Cravings: Reflect on the situations, emotions, or environments that trigger your cravings. Are there common patterns you can identify?
2. Effective Strategies: Consider which strategies have been most effective in managing your cravings. Are there specific techniques that consistently help you stay on track?
3. Challenges Faced: Reflect on the challenges you've encountered during your journey. What situations or factors tend to derail your craving control efforts?
4. Personal Growth: How have you grown as a person since you began your journey? Have you developed greater self-discipline, resilience, or self-awareness?
5. Non-Scale Wins: Reflect on the non-scale victories you've experienced. These can include improved mood, increased energy, better sleep, and enhanced overall well-being.
6. Mindset Shifts: Have you noticed any shifts in your mindset regarding food, cravings, and self-control? How have these shifts influenced your behavior?
7. Coping Mechanisms: Consider how your strategies for coping with stress, boredom, or emotions have evolved. Are you finding healthier ways to manage these triggers?
8. Long-Term Goals: Reflect on your long-term goals related to craving control. How have your initial goals evolved, and what steps are you taking to maintain your progress?

Integration of Reflection into Your Routine:

1. Set Aside Time: Dedicate regular time for reflection. This could be daily, weekly, or even monthly. The key is consistency.
2. Create a Quiet Space: Find a quiet and comfortable space where you can engage in reflection without distractions.
3. Use Prompts: Use reflective questions or prompts to guide your thoughts and insights. These prompts can help you explore different aspects of your journey.
4. Write It Down: Document your reflections in a journal or digital note. Writing helps organize your thoughts and allows you to revisit your insights later.

5. Gratitude Practice: Combine reflection with gratitude by acknowledging the positive changes and growth you've experienced on your journey.
6. Embrace Self-Compassion: Be kind to yourself during the reflection process. Avoid self-criticism and instead approach your thoughts with self-compassion.

Reflecting on your journey to craving control is a powerful tool for growth, learning, and motivation. It provides a space to celebrate your achievements, learn from your setbacks, and adapt your strategies for ongoing success. By incorporating reflection into your routine, you gain valuable insights into your triggers, behaviors, and patterns, empowering you to make informed choices that align with your health and wellness goals. Remember that your journey is ongoing, and each moment of reflection contributes to your continued progress.

•*Personal Success Stories*

The journey to weight loss is often marked by challenges, triumphs, and personal growth. Craving control plays a pivotal role in this journey, as it involves managing the intense desire for specific foods that can hinder progress. Many individuals have shared their inspiring success stories of how they conquered their cravings, achieved weight loss, and transformed their lives. These stories serve as powerful examples of determination, resilience, and the ability to overcome obstacles. In this exploration, we'll delve into personal success stories that highlight the connection between craving control and weight loss, offering insights, motivation, and practical tips for those embarking on their own journeys.

Note: These success stories are fictional but inspired by real-life experiences.

Emma's Journey from Emotional Eating to Empowerment

Emma's weight loss journey was not just about shedding pounds; it was about breaking free from emotional eating patterns that had held her captive for years. She found herself turning to food as a way to cope with stress, sadness, and even moments of happiness. Despite her initial attempts at diets and exercise, the real change happened when she focused on understanding her triggers and learning healthier ways to manage her emotions.

Emma's breakthrough came when she started practicing mindfulness. She began to recognize the moments when cravings hit and paused to ask herself whether she was truly hungry or seeking comfort. Over time, she developed alternative strategies like deep breathing, journaling, and talking to friends. As she gained more control over her emotional eating, the weight naturally started to come off.

By reflecting on her triggers and creating new coping mechanisms, Emma lost 40 pounds and gained a newfound sense of empowerment. Her success story emphasizes the importance of addressing the emotional aspects of cravings and finding healthier ways to cope.

Jake's Transformation Through Nutrient-Dense Choices

Jake's weight had always been a concern, but it wasn't until he hit his mid-30s that he decided to take his health seriously. He knew that controlling his cravings for

unhealthy foods was the key to his success. Jake adopted a strategy that revolved around making nutrient-dense choices that satisfied both his hunger and his taste buds.

Instead of completely eliminating the foods he loved, Jake focused on moderation and portion control. He would indulge in a small piece of dark chocolate or a single slice of pizza while pairing it with a balanced meal rich in lean protein, vegetables, and whole grains. By incorporating foods that were both satisfying and nutritious, he found himself less tempted by empty-calorie options.

Through consistent dedication and a commitment to smart choices, Jake lost 60 pounds over the course of a year. His story highlights the importance of balance, portion control, and the positive impact that nutrient-dense foods can have on craving control and weight loss.

Sarah's Journey from Self-Doubt to Self-Care

Sarah's weight loss journey began with a series of setbacks and self-doubt. She had tried countless diets, only to find herself giving in to cravings and feeling defeated. It wasn't until she shifted her focus from restriction to self-care that she started to see real progress.

Sarah learned to listen to her body's signals and respond with kindness. She stopped labeling foods as "good" or "bad" and embraced the concept of intuitive eating. Instead of depriving herself, she allowed herself to enjoy her favorite treats in moderation, savoring each bite mindfully.

As she developed a more positive relationship with food and her body, Sarah's cravings naturally began to diminish. She started to choose foods that made her feel energized and satisfied, rather than seeking out quick fixes. Over time, Sarah lost 50 pounds and gained a sense of self-confidence she had never experienced before.

Sarah's success story highlights the importance of self-compassion, intuitive eating, and creating a positive mindset around food and weight loss.

Mark's Transformation Through Mind-Body Connection

Mark had struggled with his weight for most of his life. He realized that his cravings were often triggered by stress and negative emotions. Determined to change, he embarked on a journey to cultivate a stronger mind-body connection.

Mark started practicing yoga and meditation, which helped him become more attuned to his body's signals. He learned to differentiate between true hunger and emotional cravings. When a craving hit, he would pause, take a few deep breaths, and ask himself whether he was truly hungry or seeking comfort.

Through consistent mindfulness practices, Mark not only gained control over his cravings but also experienced significant weight loss. He lost 80 pounds and discovered a newfound sense of balance and harmony within himself.

Mark's story underscores the power of mindfulness and the mind-body connection in managing cravings and achieving sustainable weight loss.

Personal success stories on craving control and weight loss inspire us to believe in the possibility of transformation. These stories remind us that the journey is not just about the number on the scale, but also about cultivating a healthier relationship with food, emotions, and ourselves. Whether it's overcoming emotional eating, making nutrient-dense choices, practicing self-care, or developing a mind-body connection, these stories reflect the multifaceted nature of the craving control journey. Each success story is a testament to the power of determination, self-awareness, and the willingness to embrace change for the sake of better health and well-being.

* 9 7 9 8 8 5 9 3 7 7 8 0 0 *